D0333170

99

ONE STOP DOC
Cardiology

SECC LIBRARY

T05994

One Stop Doc

Titles in the series include:

Cardiovascular System – Jonathan Aron
Editorial Advisor – Jeremy Ward

Cell and Molecular Biology – Desikan Rangarajan and David Shaw
Editorial Advisor – Barbara Moreland

Endocrine and Reproductive Systems – Caroline Jewels and Alexandra Tillett
Editorial Advisor – Stuart Milligan

Gastrointestinal System – Miruna Canagaratnam
Editorial Advisor – Richard Naftalin

Musculoskeletal System – Bassel Zebian, Wayne Lam and Rishi Aggarwal
Editorial Advisor – Alistair Hunter

Nutrition and Metabolism – Miruna Canagaratnam and David Shaw
Editorial Advisors – Barbara Moreland and Richard Naftalin

Respiratory System – Jo Dartnell and Michelle Ramsay
Editorial Advisor – John Rees

Renal and Urinary System and Electrolyte Balance – Panos Stamoulos and Spyridon Bakalis
Editorial Advisors – Alistair Hunter and Richard Naftalin

Statistics and Epidemiology – Emily Ferenczi and Nina Muirhead
Editorial Advisor – Lucy Carpenter

Immunology – Stephen Boag and Amy Sadler
Editorial Advisor – John Stewart

Gastroenterology and Renal Medicine – Reena Popat and Danielle Adebayo
Contributing Author – Thomas Chapman
Editorial Advisor – Stephen Pereira
Volume Editor – Basant Puri

ONE STOP DOC
Cardiology

Rishi Aggarwal MBBS
Graduate of Guy's, King's and St Thomas' Medical School and Senior House Officer in Accident and
Emergency Medicine, Wexham Park Hospital, Slough, UK

Emily Ferenczi BA (Cantab) BMBCh (Oxon)
FY1 Hammersmith Hospital Academic Foundation Programme, London, UK

Nina Muirhead BA (Oxon) BMBCh (Oxon)
FY1 Royal Berkshire Hospital, Reading, UK

Darrel Francis MA (Cantab) MB BChir MD MRCP
Clinical Academic in Cardiology, International Centre for Circulatory Health, Imperial College of
Science and Medicine, London and Honorary Consultant Cardiologist, St Mary's Hospital, London, UK

Volume Editor: Basant K Puri MA (Cantab) PhD MB BChir BSc (Hons) MathSci MRCPsych DipStat MMath
Professor and Consultant in Imaging and Psychiatry and Head of the Lipid Neuroscience Group,
Hammersmith Hospital, London, UK

Series Editor: Elliott Smock MBBS BSc (Hons)
FY2, University Hospital Lewisham, Lewisham, UK

Hodder Arnold
A MEMBER OF THE HODDER HEADLINE GROUP

First published in Great Britain in 2007 by
Hodder Arnold, an imprint of Hodder Education and a member of the Hodder Headline Group, an Hachette
Livre UK Company, 338 Euston Road, London NW1 3BH

http://www.hoddereducation.com

© 2007 Edward Arnold (Publishers) Ltd

All rights reserved. Apart from any use permitted under UK copyright law,
this publication may only be reproduced, stored or transmitted, in any form,
or by any means with prior permission in writing of the publishers or in the
case of reprographic production in accordance with the terms of licences
issued by the Copyright Licensing Agency. In the United Kingdom such
licences are issued by the Copyright Licensing Agency: Saffron House,
6–10 Kirby Street, London EC1N 8TS.

Whilst the advice and information in this book are believed to be true and
accurate at the date of going to press, neither the authors nor the publisher
can accept any legal responsibility or liability for any errors or omissions
that may be made. In particular, (but without limiting the generality of the
preceding disclaimer) every effort has been made to check drug dosages;
however it is still possible that errors have been missed. Furthermore,
dosage schedules are constantly being revised and new side-effects
recognized. For these reasons the reader is strongly urged to consult the
drug companies' printed instructions before administering any of the drugs
recommended in this book.

British Library Cataloguing in Publication Data
A catalogue record for this book is available from the British Library

Library of Congress Cataloging-in-Publication Data
A catalog record for this book is available from the Library of Congress

ISBN 978 0340 925577

1 2 3 4 5 6 7 8 9 10

Commissioning Editor: Sara Purdy
Project Editor: Jane Tod
Production Controller: Lindsay Smith
Cover Design: Amina Dudhia
Indexer: Indexing Specialists (UK) Ltd

Typeset in 10/12pt Adobe Garamond/Akzidenz GroteskBE by Servis Filmsetting Ltd, Manchester
Printed and bound in Spain

What do you think about this book? Or any other Hodder Arnold title?
Please visit our website at **www.hoddereducation.com**

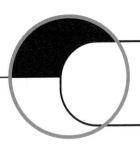

CONTENTS

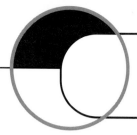

PREFACE

From the Series Editor, Elliott Smock

Are you ready to face your looming exams? If you have done loads of work, then congratulations; we hope this opportunity to practice SAQs, EMQs, MCQs and Problem-based Questions on every part of the core curriculum will help you consolidate what you've learnt and improve your exam technique. If you don't feel ready, don't panic – the One Stop Doc series has all the answers you need to catch up and pass.

There are only a limited number of questions an examiner can throw at a beleaguered student and this text can turn that to your advantage. By getting straight into the heart of the core questions that come up year after year and by giving you the model answers you need this book will arm you with the knowledge to succeed in your exams. Broken down into logical sections, you can learn all the important facts you need to pass without having to wade through tons of different textbooks when you simply don't have the time. All questions presented here are 'core'; those of the highest importance have been highlighted to allow even sharper focus if time for revision is running out. In addition, to allow you to organize your revision efficiently, questions have been grouped by topic, with answers supported by detailed integrated explanations.

On behalf of all the One Stop Doc authors I wish you the very best of luck in your exams and hope these books serve you well!

From the Authors, Rishi Aggarwal, Emily Ferenczi and Nina Muirhead

The horizons of cardiology are expanding at an astonishing rate with the use of medicines such as statins, thrombolytics and antiplatelet antibodies; interventions such as percutaneous angioplasty and surgery to implant artificial hearts, to name but a few recent developments. Patients with congenital cardiac defects are now living well into adulthood, creating a new subspecialty of 'adult congenital cardiac disease'. For those interested in public health, an increase in understanding of the importance of primary prevention and early modification of cardiac risk factors has led to a plethora of new guidelines and targets for cardiac care in the community.

The WHO has said that by 2020, the leading cause of global disease burden will be ischaemic heart disease. As a result, every doctor must expect to face patients with cardiological problems, no matter what specialty they eventually decide to pursue. For this reason it is essential to have a thorough understanding of the basic principles of cardiac physiology, many of which are based on simple laws of physics – pressures, resistances and volumes or electrical currents, voltages and conductance. In this book we aim to inform and to inspire medical students by providing a simple but comprehensive summary of clinical cardiology with questions and explanations side by side to make learning relevant to the clinical practice that they will be witnessing on a daily basis.

We would like to thank Dr Darrel Francis, Professor Basant Puri, our friends and families, and Hodder Arnold, for making this book possible.

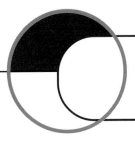

ABBREVIATIONS

2D	Two-dimensional
ABC	Airway, breathing, circulation
ACE	Angiotensin-converting enzyme
ACS	Acute coronary syndrome
ADH	Anti-diuretic hormone
AF	Atrial fibrillation
AIDS	Acquired immune deficiency syndrome
AR	Aortic regurgitation
ASD	Atrial septal defect
ASO	Antistreptolysin-O
AV	Atrioventricular
AVNRT	Atrioventricular node re-entry tachycardia
AVRT	Atrioventricular re-entry tachycardia
b.d.	Twice daily
BM	Boehringer Mannheim (test)
BMI	Body mass index
BP	Blood pressure
bpm	Beats per minute
CABG	Coronary artery bypass graft
CCU	Coronary care unit
CK	Creatine kinase
CK-MB	Creatinine kinase, myocardial isoenzyme
CNS	Central nervous system
COPD	Chronic obstructive pulmonary disease
CPAP	Continuous positive airway pressure
CPR	Cardiopulmonary resuscitation
CRP	C-reactive protein
CT	Computed tomography
CXR	Chest radiography
DC	Direct current
DVLA	Driver and Vehicle Licensing Agency
DVT	Deep vein thrombosis
ECG	Electrocardiography
ESR	Erythrocyte sedimentation rate
ETT	Exercise treadmill test
FBC	Full blood count
GP	General practitioner
GTN	Glyceryl trinitrate
HDL	High-density lipoprotein
HIV	Human immunodeficiency virus
HOCM	Hypertrophic obstructive cardiomyopathy
ICS	Intercostal space
ICU	Intensive care unit
IHD	Ischaemic heart disease
INR	International Normalized Ratio
ISMN	Isosorbide mononitrate
IV	Intravenous
JVP	Jugular venous pressure
LA	Left atrium
LAD	Left anterior descending
LBBB	Left bundle branch block
LCA	Left coronary artery
LCx	Left circumflex
LDH	Lactate dehydrogenase
LDL	Low-density lipoprotein
LMWH	Low molecular weight heparin
LV	Left ventricle
LVH	Left ventricular hypertrophy
MI	Myocardial infarction
MR	Mitral regurgitation
MRI	Magnetic resonance imaging
NSAID	Non-steroidal anti-inflammatory drug
NSTEMI	Non-ST elevation myocardial infarction
PCI	Percutaneous coronary intervention
PE	Pulmonary embolism
PET	Positron emission tomography
POBA	'Plain old balloon angioplasty'
PTCA	Percutaneous transluminal coronary angioplasty
RA	Right atrium
RBBB	Right bundle branch block
RCA	Right coronary artery
RV	Right ventricle
RVH	Right ventricular hypertrophy
S1	First heart sound
S2	Second heart sound
S3	Third heart sound

S4	Fourth heart sound	**TB**	Tuberculosis
SA	Sinoatrial	**TOE**	Transoesophageal echocardiography
SK	Streptrokinase	**tPA**	Tissue plasminogen activator
SLE	Systemic lupus erythematosus	**U&Es**	Urea and electrolytes
SSRI	Selective serotonin re-uptake inhibitor	**VF**	Ventricular fibrillation
		VSD	Ventricular septal defect
STEMI	ST elevation myocardial infarction	**VT**	Ventricular tachycardia
SVT	Supraventricular tachycardia	**ZN**	Ziehl–Neelsen

SECTION (**1**) # HISTORY AND EXAMINATION

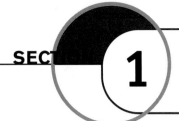

1

HISTORY AND EXAMINATION

1. Separate the following symptoms/signs into those associated with (i) right-sided heart failure and (ii) left-sided heart failure (options may be used more than once)

    a. Orthopnoea
    b. Ascites
    c. Paroxysmal nocturnal dyspnoea
    d. Peripheral oedema
    e. Exertional dyspnoea

2. Case study

While working in an A&E department, your registrar asks you to clerk a 57-year-old man who has been referred by a local GP. Reading the referral letter, you note that the patient has been complaining of recent onset central chest pain.

    a. Using the information given, calculate this man's body mass index. What does this value mean?
    b. What are the key points to elicit from this man's history to establish his risk of coronary artery disease?

The patient goes on to describe a smoking history of approximately 25 cigarettes per day over a period of 40 years.

    c. Convert his cigarette consumption into pack-years

EXPLANATION: CARDIOVASCULAR HISTORY

History of presenting complaint

- Chest pain (site, character, radiation, precipitating factors, duration and relieving factors)
- Syncope
- Palpitations (duration, frequency of episodes).

Symptoms suggestive of right-sided failure	Symptoms suggestive of left-sided heart failure
Exertional dyspnoea	Exertional dyspnoea (acute/chronic), exacerbating factors (e.g. lying down), exercise tolerance, association with cough, productive of sputum – colour/wheeze/haemoptysis
Abdominal swelling suggestive of ascites	Paroxysmal nocturnal dyspnoea (acute shortness of breath that wakes patient and is relieved by sitting up)
Ankle swelling suggestive of peripheral oedema	Orthopnoea (inability to lie flat – how many pillows required to sleep?)

Past medical history

- Cardiac ischaemia (angina/previous MI)
- Stroke, peripheral vascular disease
- Rheumatic fever
- Hypertension
- Previous cardiac investigations
- Previous treatment: medication/CABG/angioplasty.

Coronary artery disease risk factors (2b)

- Family history of MI before the age of 55 years in a first-degree relative
- Smoker (1 pack-year = smoking 20 cigarettes per day for 1 year)
- Hypertension, diabetes mellitus, hypercholesterolaemia
- Obesity: **BMI** = body mass in kilograms/(height in meters)^2 (underweight ≤18.5; normal weight 18.5–24.9; overweight 25–29.9; obesity ≥30); it is also important to take fat distribution into account – abdominal or truncal obesity is associated with hyperinsulinaemia, hypertriglyceridaemia, reduced concentrations of HDL cholesterol and hypertension)
- Gender (males are at greater risk of coronary heart disease)
- Ethnicity (increased coronary heart disease risk in those from the Asian subcontinent).

Social history

- Alcohol intake in units (recommended consumption 21 units per week for men and 14 units per week for women).

Medications/allergies

- Previous treatment with streptokinase (thrombolytic agent) for MI. See also the explanation on treatments (see page 77).

Answers

1. (i) b, d, e; (ii) a, c, e
2. a – 30.1, indicating that he is obese, b – See explanation, c – 50 pack-years

3. (a) What is the name given to the clinical sign that is depicted in this series of diagrams? (b) State two cardiac-related conditions that may cause it

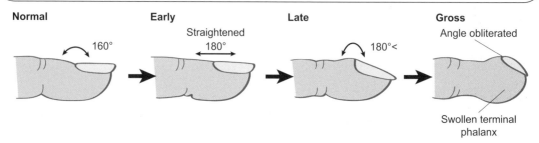

Normal   **Early**   **Late**   **Gross**
                Straightened   Angle obliterated
160°   180°   180°<

Swollen terminal
phalanx

4. The drawing on the left shows a thumb from a patient with chronic iron deficiency. (a) What clinical sign does this patient have? (b) Name another cardiac-related condition that you may expect this sign to present in. (c) Name the clinical signs labelled A and B

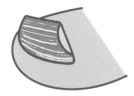   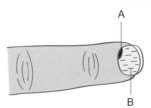

A

B

5. Hypertensive retinal changes are graded to signify the level of retinopathy. Match each of the changes below with the appropriate grade of disease in which it would FIRST be seen

Options

A. Grade 1   1. Cotton wool spots
B. Grade 2   2. Irregular points of focal constriction
C. Grade 3   3. Flame haemorrhages
D. Grade 4   4. Hard exudates
E. Grade 5   5. Minimal arteriolar narrowing
                          6. Papilloedema

6. The dusky blue discoloration of a patient's lips characteristically indicates central cyanosis. However, what is the minimum level of deoxygenated blood that must be present for this clinical sign to be apparent? Choose the most appropriate answer from the options provided

a. 50 g/L   b. 5 mg/dL   c. 0.5 g/dL   d. 5 g/L   e. 5 dL

EXPLANATION: SIGNS ON EXAMINATION (I)

Hands

- Temperature
- **Capillary refill time**: apply pressure on nail bed for 5 seconds, after which it should resume normal colour in <2 seconds; this is a crude test to establish the degree of peripheral tissue perfusion or dehydration
- **Peripheral cyanosis**: resulting from peripheral vascular disease or poor cardiac output
- **Koilonychia**: (spoon-shaped nails) may indicate established iron deficiency or ischaemic heart disease
- **Cardiac-related digital clubbing**: may be the result of congenital heart disease, bacterial endocarditis or atrial myxoma
- **Splinter haemorrhages**: linear haemorrhages in the nail bed, parallel to the length of the nail, that can present in endocarditis

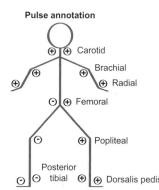

Pulse annotation

- **Osler's nodes**: painful, pink, pea-sized papules over the finger pads; associated with bacterial endocarditis
- **Janeway lesions**: non-tender maculae on the palms and soles that are red to bluish-red in colour; also associated with endocarditis
- **Nicotine staining**: characteristically around index and middle fingers and supported by presence on teeth.

Pulse

- **Radial pulse**: note rate, rhythm (sinus/irregularly irregular), volume, character (e.g. slow rising/collapsing), radioradial delay, radiofemoral delay
- **Bradycardia**: <60 bpm
- **Tachycardia**: >100 bpm.

Eyes

- **Xanthelasma**: cholesterol deposits located around the eyes
- **Conjunctival pallor**: present when haemoglobin is <**10 g/dL**

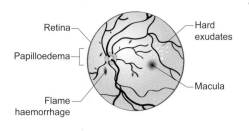

- **Hypertensive retinopathy**: vessels at the back of the eye are particularly sensitive to hypertension; such changes are graded as follows

    Grade 1: minimal arteriolar narrowing

    Grade 2: marked arteriolar narrowing with irregular points of focal constriction

    Grade 3: grade 2 plus retinal (flame) haemorrhages, cotton wool spots and/or hard exudates

    Grade 4: grade 3 plus swelling (papilloedema) of the optic disc.

Lips and tongue

- Dusky blue discoloration indicates central cyanosis – at least **5 g/dL** of deoxygenated haemoglobin in arterial blood.

Answers

3. a – Digital clubbing, b – Congenital heart disease, bacterial endocarditis or atrial myxoma
4. a – Koilonychia, b – Ischaemic heart disease, c – A, Nail fold infarction, B, Splinter haemorrhages
5. 1 – C, 2 – B, 3 – C, 4 – C, 5 – A, 6 – D (grade 4 most severe)
6. a (conventionally given in g/dL)

7. Concerning the JVP, true or false?

    a. The jugular venous pressure is measured with the patient in a recumbent position
    b. The jugular venous pressure reflects pressure changes in the left atrium
    c. The jugular venous pressure is taken to be the vertical distance (in cm) from the sternal angle to the top of the jugular venous pulsation
    d. A jugular venous pressure of $3\,cmH_2O$ is considered to be normal
    e. The jugular venous pulsation is not normally visible in the neck

8. **Describe the clinical characteristics of the carotid pulse that allow it to be differentiated from the jugular venous pulse**

9. **Describe the physiological basis for hepatojugular reflux and its relationship with JVP**

10. **Describe the physiological basis for Kussmaul's sign and its relationship with JVP**

11. **Kussmaul's sign is most likely be seen in which ONE of the following conditions?**

    a. Gastric reflux
    b. Cardiac tamponade
    c. Superior vena cava obstruction
    d. Tricuspid regurgitation
    e. Right-sided heart failure

12. **True or false? The following conditions are likely to cause elevated JVP**

    a. Pregnancy
    b. Pulmonary embolism
    c. Blood transfusion
    d. Retrosternal thyroid goitre
    e. Emphysema

EXPLANATION: SIGNS ON EXAMINATION II

The **JVP** should be assessed with the patient lying at an angle of 45° to the horizontal and in good light. View the right side of the neck for a double-wave pulsation with each heartbeat. If this is present, you are observing a column of blood in the internal jugular vein. Its upward and downward movement reflects pressure change in the right atrium. Normally, this is less than $3\,cmH_2O$ and is not visible, as it lies just beneath the right clavicle. The value is measured by taking the vertical distance from the sternal angle to the top of the jugular venous pulsation. A pressure exceeding $9\,cmH_2O$ at the RA (i.e. >3–4 cm above the sternal angle) is considered to be raised and consequently abnormal.

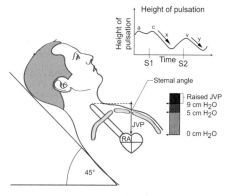

It is essential that you learn and understand how to differentiate jugular pulsation from the carotid pulse **(8)**, as they both present in the neck. Most importantly, the jugular pulsation is non-palpable, rises when pressure is applied to the liver (as this causes more blood to be expelled into the right side of the heart – hepatojugular reflux) and falls when the patient is upright. The JVP can be stopped by gently pressing against the neck to occlude the internal jugular vein. The carotid pulse is a single pulsation per cardiac cycle that does not vary with hepatojugular reflux, posture or respiration. It is palpable, but not readily occludable.

Components of a normal jugular venous pulse

a wave	RA contraction
c wave	RV contracts causing closure and then bulging of tricuspid valve
x descent	Atrial relaxation
v wave	Ventricular contraction: filling of RA
y descent	Ventricular relaxation: drop in RA pressure as tricuspid valve reopens

Hepatojugular reflux **(9)** is a useful test in patients with right-sided heart failure, as hepatomegaly may occur in right-sided heart failure and venous congestion. The patient lies down in the same position as for JVP measurement, keeping the mouth open and breathing normally (to prevent the Valsalva manoeuvre, which may give a false-positive test). Moderate pressure is applied over the middle of the abdomen for 30–60 seconds. The test is positive if the JVP increases by at least 3 cm and is maintained during the period of compression.

The physiological norm is for the JVP to rise during expiration and fall on inspiration (along with intrathoracic pressure). Kussmaul's sign is the paradoxical finding of a rising JVP on inspiration **(10)**; the classical differential diagnosis is constrictive pericarditis, cardiac tamponade or pericardial effusion.

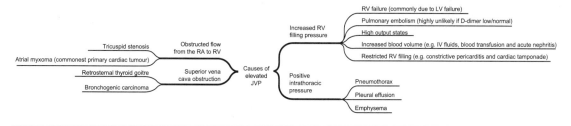

Answers

7. F F T T T
8. See explanation
9. See explanation
10. See explanation
11. b
12. T T T T T

13. Match each of the cases described with the most appropriate cardiac defect/murmur listed below. You may use the options more than once or not at all

Options

A. Tricuspid stenosis
B. Benign murmur
C. Austin Flint murmur
D. Mitral stenosis
E. Pulmonary regurgitation
F. Venous hum

G. Patent ductus arteriosus
H. Atrial septal defect
I. Aortic stenosis
J. Mitral regurgitation
K. Ventricular septal defect

1. A 6-year-old boy has an ejection systolic murmur
2. A 27-year-old man has a 'rumbling' mid-diastolic murmur. The patient gives a history of rheumatic fever in his teens
3. A 50-year-old man has a murmur that starts in systole and ends in diastole. It is restricted to the neck and is not audible when the patient is supine
4. A 40-year-old woman has an early diastolic murmur. It is audible with the bell of a stethoscope and is described as a soft, high-pitched, 'blowing' sound. Her pulse is of normal character
5. An 8-year-old girl has a continuous murmur that has a 'machinery' quality. It is heard well just below the left clavicle
6. An 95-year-old man had an early diastolic murmur for several years, but recently this has changed into a mid-late diastolic 'rumbling'

14. Match each of the systemic diseases below with the murmur with which it is characteristically associated (you may use the same answer more than once or not at all)

Options

A. Aortic stenosis
B. Aortic regurgitation
C. Mitral stenosis
D. Mitral regurgitation
E. Pulmonary stenosis
F. Pulmonary regurgitation
G. Ejection systolic murmur due to high cardiac output

1. Behçet's disease
2. Down's syndrome
3. Marfan's syndrome
4. Noonan's syndrome
5. Thyrotoxicosis
6. Fallot's tetralogy

15. The bell of a stethoscope allows one to appreciate the audible characteristics of low-pitched sounds. State the two murmurs that require use of the bell

S2, second heart sound; ICS, intercostal space; AV, atrioventricular

EXPLANATION: MURMURS AND THE CARDIAC CYCLE

Mid-systolic/ejection systolic: These murmurs begin after the opening of the aortic and pulmonary valves, while blood is being ejected from the ventricles into the great vessels. The intensity rises to the mid-point of systole and then falls before S2. **Pulmonary stenosis**: commonly congenital, the murmur is associated with Noonan's syndrome and Fallot's tetralogy. It is loudest at the second ICS. **Associated with atrial septal defect**: due to high pressure in the pulmonary artery. **Associated with anaemia, pregnancy and thyrotoxicosis**: due to the state of high cardiac output. **Benign murmur**: a normal and frequent occurrence in children.

Pansystolic: These are murmurs due to sustained pressure differences across a defective valve or septum, throughout systole. **Mitral regurgitation. Tricuspid regurgitation**: prominent over the lower left sternal edge or even the xiphisternum. It may be confused with mitral regurgitation as it frequently radiates to the apex, but when heard during inspiration the murmur is significantly louder. **Ventricular septal defect**: a relatively loud murmur that is prominent over the lower left sternal edge.

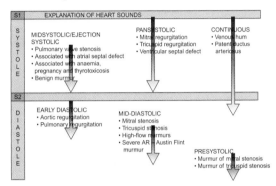

Continuous: These murmurs begin during systole, but follow through into diastole. **Venous hum**: usually loudest in the neck. It is caused by high blood flow in the jugular veins. It may disappear completely when the patient is flat. **Patent ductus arteriosus**: heard when blood passes from the high-pressure aorta into the lower pressure of the pulmonary artery. Is loudest at the left second ICS or below the left clavicle and has a 'machinery' quality.

Early diastolic: These begin after the closure of the aortic or pulmonary valves. There is a regurgitant jet of blood past these valves to their respective ventricles. A soft, high-pitched 'blowing' is audible, accentuated when the patient is sitting forwards in full expiration. **Aortic regurgitation. Pulmonary regurgitation**: a rare murmur that is best heard over the third or fourth ICS below the aortic valve. Unlike aortic regurgitation, it is not associated with a collapsing peripheral pulse.

Mid-diastolic: These are the result of blood flow through the AV valves. Hence, they are audible some time after S2. **Mitral stenosis. Tricuspid stenosis**: rare; many cases are due to rheumatic heart disease and it is common to find coexisting mitral stenosis. The murmur is described as 'scratchy' and is best heard over the lower left sternal edge with the bell of a stethoscope and the patient inspiring. **High-flow murmurs**: due to high blood flow across the AV valves. Typical examples include those associated with mitral regurgitation, ventricular septal defect and patent ductus arteriosus or even atrial septal defect. **Severe aortic regurgitation**: Austin Flint murmur.

Presystolic: Best heard over the left lower sternal border and are heightened by inspiration. **Murmur of mitral stenosis**: best heard with the patient lying in a left lateral position. Murmur of **tricuspid stenosis**: produced as blood is forced through narrowed mitral or tricuspid valves during atrial systole.

Answers

13. 1 – B, 2 – D (tricuspid stenosis may coexist, but extremely difficult to detect on auscultation), 3 – F, 4 – E, 5 – G, 6 – C
14. 1 – B, 2 – D, 3 – B, 4 – E, 5 – G, 6 – E
15. Mitral stenosis and tricuspid stenosis

EXPLANATION: LEFT-SIDED HEART MURMURS

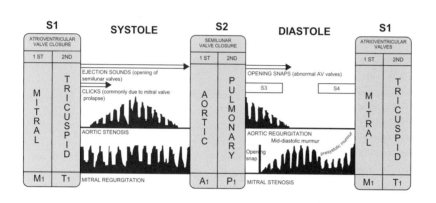

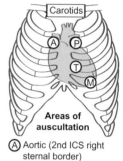

Carotids

Areas of auscultation

(A) Aortic (2nd ICS right sternal border)
(P) Pulmonary (2nd ICS left sternal border)
(T) Tricuspid (4th ICS left sternal border)
(M) Mitral/apex (5th mid-clavicular line)

Aortic stenosis: A characteristically 'harsh'-sounding, crescendo-decrescendo **ejection systolic murmur**. It is best heard over the **aortic area** and can be **traced into the neck**. The LV contracting against the stenotic valve becomes pressure overloaded and **LVH** ensues. The pulse created is also **slow rising** and of **low volume**. Common causes: congenital, rheumatic heart disease and age-acquired calcification/fibrosis of the valve or chordae tendinae.

Aortic regurgitation: An **early diastolic 'blowing'** murmur, created as blood passes back across the valve. It is best heard over the **pulmonary area**, and the backflow results in a **collapsing pulse** within the aorta. In diastole, the LV is receiving backflowing (past the aortic valve) as well as forward-flowing blood (past the mitral valve). In time, this pressure causes **LVH**. Additionally, as the ventricle is filling up faster than normal, the mitral valve is forced to close earlier; this can give a 'rumbling' late diastolic murmur (**Austin Flint murmur**).

Mitral stenosis: A **mid-diastolic 'rumbling'**, the duration of which is increased with worsening disease. Its **low pitch** requires the bell of a stethoscope and overall it is **loudest over the apex (mitral area), with extension into the left axilla**. It is commonly accompanied by an **opening snap**, a **presystolic murmur** and a **loud S1**. Chronic disease leads to **left atrial hypertrophy** (predisposing to **atrial fibrillation**) together with **pulmonary hypertension**. Ninety-nine per cent of patients have had previous episodes of acute **rheumatic fever** and present later, in their 20–30s, with dyspnoea secondary to **pulmonary congestion**.

Mitral regurgitation: A **high-pitched pansystolic murmur** heard best at the apex, especially with the patient in the left lateral position with the breath held in expiration. Typically, it radiates to the left axilla and the left infrascapular region, Patients with mild disease are **usually asymptomatic**, as compensatory mechanisms result in **LV dilatation and LVH**. Often S1 is soft and S2 is widely split.

ICS, intercostal space; S1, first heart sound; S2, second heart sound; S3, third heart sound; S4 fourth heart sound; LVH, left ventricular hypertrophy

SECTION 2

SYMPTOMS

2 SYMPTOMS

1. **For each patient, select the most likely diagnosis for their chest pain from the options provided**

Options

   A. Angina
   B. Aortic dissection
   C. Costochondritis
   D. Gastro-oesophageal reflux
   E. Myocardial infarction
   F. Pleurisy
   G. Pneumonia
   H. Pulmonary embolism
   I. Pneumothorax

   1. A 37-year-old man had fever and malaise for 10 days; for the last 12 hours, he has had severe left-sided chest pain that is exacerbated by movement or respiration
   2. A 45-year-old man complains of heartburn and acid brash, worse in the mornings
   3. A 54-year-old smoker presents with shortness of breath, heavy perspiration and central chest pain of 1 hour's duration
   4. A 60-year-old diabetic presents with a sudden onset of left jaw and throat pain, lasting 5 minutes and relieved by sublingual nitrates
   5. A 60-year-old hypertensive man presents with sudden, tearing central chest pain radiating between the shoulder blades

2. **A 62-year-old man presents to your A&E department. He is extremely distressed and complains of sudden-onset chest pain. He is in no state to give a thorough history**

   a. Using the information provided, name four life-threatening cardiovascular conditions that this man may be presenting with
   b. Name two non-cardiac conditions that could present in a similar manner
   c. List the three most important investigations that would help you to evaluate this man's chest pain

EXPLANATION: CHEST PAIN

This is a common complaint that may be experienced by patients with an underlying cardiac pathology. Equally, it is a non-specific symptom that can be the result of a range of serious as well as relatively benign conditions. In addition to examining the patient, great importance is placed on a good history, focusing on the characteristics of the pain and any other associated symptoms. First-line investigations, particularly in the A&E environment, should include the following: **serial ECG**, **CXR** and **cardiac enzymes/troponin T**. Six major causes of chest pain are outlined in the table below.

	Myocardial ischaemias*	Musculo-skeletal	Gastro-oesophageal	Pleuritic	Pericarditis	Aortic dissection
Site	Retrosternal	Localized to chest wall	Central chest	Localized to chest wall	Retrosternal	Central chest
Character	Dull ache, constriction, heavy, crushing	Aching, pricking, sharp	Burning	Sharp, pleuritic	Sharp, sore	Tearing
Radiation	Left arm, shoulders, neck, jaw	None	Back, shoulder blades, throat, abdomen	Shoulders, back	Tip of left shoulder	Between shoulder blades
Duration	MI >30 minutes, Angina <10 minutes	Constant	Constant or intermittent	Constant	Constant	Constant
Precipitating/ relieving factors	Worse on exercise or stress, cold, after food; improves with nitrates/rest	Worse on movement, local palpation and respiration	Relieved by food or milk and worse in the morning	Worse on movement and inspiration	Worse on inspiration and lying flat; easier on expiration and sitting forwards	Nil
Associated symptoms	Sweating, nausea, breathless-ness	Bruising with a history of trauma	Dysphagia, water brash, acid reflux, relation to food	Dyspnoea, cough fever, haemoptysis	Fever, breathlessness	Collapse, sweating, hypotension, chest pain from myocardial ischaemia

*20 per cent of patients with confirmed MI do not have a history of chest pain (generally the elderly and those with diabetes)

Answers

1. 1 – F (duration of symptoms makes pneumonia unlikely), 2 – D, 3 – E, 4 – A, 5 – B
2. a – MI, aortic dissection, unstable angina, pulmonary embolism, b – Tension pneumothorax, oesophageal rupture, c – ECG, CXR, cardiac enzymes/troponin T

Case study: dyspnoea

Mrs Crane, a 66-year-old woman known to suffer from heart failure, attends your cardiology clinic. Currently, her medical treatment includes diuretics. Over the last few weeks she has become progressively short of breath, so much so that she has found herself breathless during simple daily activities: 'I get up in the morning, walk to the bathroom and find myself gasping for air.'

3. How can we classify this woman's symptomatic heart failure and where does she fall on this scale?

4. The following statements concerning exertional dyspnoea are true

   a. It does not occur in healthy individuals
   b. It may be caused by a reduction in oxygen saturation
   c. Myocardial infarction is the commonest cause
   d. Breathlessness is caused by a reduction in cardiac preload leading to the formation of pulmonary oedema

5. Mrs Crane goes on to explain that she requires four pillows to sleep at night, as lying flat can put her out of breath. What is the term given to her sleeping difficulties?

6. (a) Name two long-term complications of right-sided heart failure. (b) How may these complications compound Mrs Crane's breathing difficulties?

7. Mrs Crane describes a frightening incident that occurred last night: 'I must have been sleeping for about an hour. Suddenly, I woke up very short of breath and struggled to the window, to get some air.' What is she describing and why does it happen?

EXPLANATION: DYSPNOEA (BREATHLESSNESS)

Dyspnoea: This is an **uncomfortable awareness of one's own breathing**. It may occur acutely (e.g. MI) or over a longer period of time in chronic disease.

Exertional dyspnoea: Generally, physiological breathlessness on exertion is normal and represents insufficient tissue oxygenation. It is termed **pathological (exertional) dyspnoea** when it occurs at a lower level of exertion than would normally be expected. **Left-sided heart failure** is the commonest cause. When this side of the heart is functioning suboptimally, back pressure on the pulmonary circulation is increased, resulting in pooling of fluid in the lungs (pulmonary oedema) and ultimately impaired oxygenation of the blood. Also, as a result of neurohormonal imbalances and physical detraining, the peripheral vasculature and musculature deteriorate in quality, and receptors in the limbs trigger the sensation of dyspnoea at lower workloads.

Orthopnoea: This is the name given to **dyspnoea experienced when a patient is recumbent** (lying down). The recumbent position increases venous return and adds to the already congested pulmonary venous system, consequently worsening **pulmonary oedema** and reducing lung compliance.

Right-sided heart failure normally follows left-sided failure, due to the chronic effects of raised pulmonary venous pressure. It is also associated with the complications of ascites and hepatomegaly, which compound orthopnoeic dyspnoea by raising the diaphragm further into the thoracic cavity, thereby reducing vital capacity.

Paroxysmal nocturnal dyspnoea: This can be a very frightening experience for people suffering **pulmonary oedema (7)**. As they sleep, their awareness of breathing and sleeping position are reduced. From time to time, they lie in a position that precipitates further pulmonary oedema (e.g. lying flat), which induce acute episodes of dyspnoea; patients often describe attacks of breathlessness that force them to sit up and struggle at the bedside 'to get air'.

In patients with heart disease, functional dyspnoea is classified by the New York Heart Association in the following manner.

Class	Degree of breathlessness
Class I	No breathlessness
Class II	Breathlessness on severe exertion
Class III	Breathlessness on mild exertion
Class IV	Breathlessness at rest

ANSWERS

3. New York Heart Association classification of heart failure, class III
4. F T F F
5. Orthopnoea
6. a – Ascites and hepatomegaly, b – ↓ Vital capacity
7. Paroxysmal nocturnal dyspnoea. See explanation

8. (a) Define presyncope. (b) Define syncope. (c) Describe the role of Holter monitoring and memory loop recorders in gathering information about presyncopal or syncopal episodes. In what circumstances should each technique be used?

9. For each patient, select the most likely diagnosis for his/her syncope-related episodes from the options provided

Options

A. Supraventricular tachycardia
B. Atrial fibrillation
C. 2:1 atrioventricular block
D. Sinus rhythm
E. Postural syncope (orthostatic hypotension)
F. Carotid sinus syndrome
G. Severe aortic stenosis
H. Hypertrophic obstructive cardiomyopathy
I. Micturition syncope
J. Vasovagal syncope
K. Stokes–Adams attack
L. Autonomic dysfunction

1. A 23-year-old female medical student has had several episodes in which she loses consciousness while at home. She explains that she feels hot and clammy just before each episode. She will be sitting her finals next week
2. A 60-year-old woman with the following rhythm strip, which reverts to sinus rhythm after carotid sinus massage

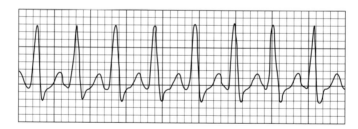

3. A 74-year-old man has recently been feeling 'dizzy', particularly during the day. He saw his GP two weeks ago about 'swollen legs'. He believes that the GP increased one of his normal medications and he has been passing urine with increased frequency
4. A 60-year-old man explains that he felt light-headed several days ago. At the time he was writing a letter and dropped his pen. When he went to pick it up (while seated), he felt as though he was about to faint
5. An 18-year-old woman loses consciousness while out running. Her ECG taken in the local A&E department shows LV hypertrophy and broad Q waves. She is awaiting echocardiography
6. A 62-year-old man who is a known alcoholic complains of passing out while on the toilet

HOCM, hypertrophic obstructive cardiomyopathy

EXPLANATION: CARDIOVASCULAR-RELATED SYNCOPE

Presyncope describes weakness or cognitive symptoms without loss of consciousness, whereas **syncope** is a sudden, transient loss of consciousness **(8)**. Victims lose muscle tone and become unresponsive momentarily, making a full recovery within seconds to minutes. The causes are derived from three main areas: **cardiovascular**, **neurological** and **cerebrovascular**. All episodes are ultimately the result of inadequate perfusion of the brain, which is dependent on cardiac output, arterial blood pressure and resistance of the cerebral circulation. In one-half of all cases, a diagnosis is made after a careful history and physical examination, combined with ECG. ECG is helpful in identifying abnormalities of the rhythm, conduction or morphology of heart electrical activity. ECG recordings from daily episodes may be obtained through continuous **24-hour ambulatory monitoring (Holter monitoring)**. **Memory loop recorders** are helpful for infrequent episodes; patients can initiate monitoring when they experience symptoms suggestive of a 'spell' **(8)**. More recently, implantable monitors have been made available for those who need chronic monitoring of heart function. A flow diagram at the end of this section (see page 20) outlines the work-up for syncopal episodes. Common cardiovascular causes are explained below.

Arrhythmias: In **supraventricular and ventricular tachycardias**, the heart rate may exceed 180 bpm. This provides insufficient time for adequate ventricular filling and cardiac output falls dramatically. In contrast, **Stokes–Adams attacks** involve an extreme drop in the pulse rate as a result of underlying heart block, where prolonged attacks may lead to convulsions and even death.

Postural syncope (orthostatic hypotension): Patients may experience dizziness on sitting or standing that is followed by syncope. In such cases, the normal vasoconstrictive mechanisms that prevent blood pooling in the legs fail (e.g. **elderly**, **autonomic dysfunction** associated with **diabetic neuropathy**) or there is underlying hypotension, which increases susceptibility to such attacks (e.g. **dehydration**, **blood loss**, **diuretics**, **antihypertensive drugs**).

Carotid sinus syndrome: In this condition, presyncope or syncope may be precipitated by any manoeuvre that stimulates the **carotid sinus** (e.g. head turning); a sudden drop in heart rate and reflex hypotension follow. It is a rare finding below the age of 50 years.

Syncope on exertion: This **always requires investigation**, because it may be the only symptom preceding sudden cardiac death. It is a characteristic feature of **severe aortic stenosis** and **HOCM**, where the heart is unable to increase cardiac output in the face of the increased demands placed on it.

Micturition syncope: This occurs in men suffering **nocturia**, frequently after consumption of alcohol.

Vasomotor/vasovagal syncope or simple faint: This is when a patient experiences a brief loss of consciousness, preceded by a sense of anticipation in which there is an increase and then a sudden decrease in sympathetic tone, blood pressure and pulse. The victim generally recovers after a few minutes spent in a supine position. **Tilt testing** attempts to provoke vasovagal syncope by strapping the patient onto a table and gradually elevating it from flat to near-upright. It is often used in patients with recurrent syncope who have no structural cardiac abnormality and in whom Holter monitoring has been normal. It aims to identify patients with a prominent fall in heart rate before syncope who may benefit from implantation of a pacemaker.

Answers

8. See explanation
9. 1 – J, 2 – A, 3 – E (diuretic treatment), 4 – F, 5 – H, 6 – I

10. The following may result in peripheral oedema. True or false?

a. Hypoalbuminaemia
b. Sodium retention
c. Hepatic cirrhosis
d. Vena caval obstruction
e. Heart failure

11. Best response. Peripheral oedema is clinically apparent when extracellular volume has risen by at least

a. 5 per cent
b. 10 per cent
c. 20 per cent
d. 40 per cent
e. 50 per cent

12. Short answer question. Concerning peripheral oedema

What is the main factor that determines the bodily distribution of such fluid?
Why may it be termed pitting oedema?
Describe the physiological processes that lead to its formation in cardiac failure

ADH, anti-diuertic hormone

EXPLANATION: PERIPHERAL OEDEMA

Peripheral oedema is the **accumulation of fluid within the interstitial tissues**. It is clinically apparent when there is at least a **10–15 per cent** rise in the extracellular volume. It is commonly the result of congestive heart failure. Other causes include:

- **Hypoalbuminaemia**
- **Sodium retention**
- **Hepatic cirrhosis**
- **Vena caval obstruction.**

The diagram below shows how cardiac failure results in peripheral oedema **(12)**.

The peripheral distribution of the fluid is determined largely by **gravity**. In mobile patients, fluid begins to pool around the **ankles**. Bed-bound patients initially acquire fluid at the **sacrum**; it subsequently accumulates in first the lower and then the upper limbs. Temporary dimples or pits are formed when pressure is applied to these areas **(12)**, giving rise to the term pitting oedema. Peripheral oedema is a late manifestation of cardiac failure, and patients are likely to have fluid in other places first (pleural effusion and/or pericardial effusion). Treatment strategies are described on page 107.

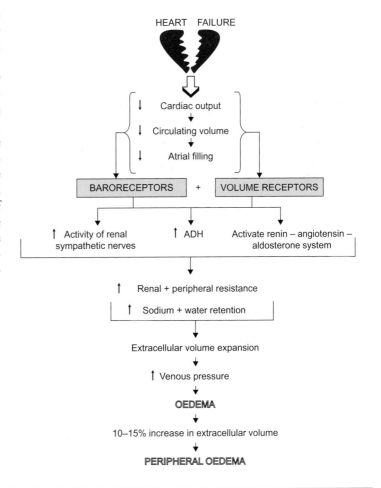

A PATHWAY FOR THE EVALUATION OF SYNCOPAL EPISODES

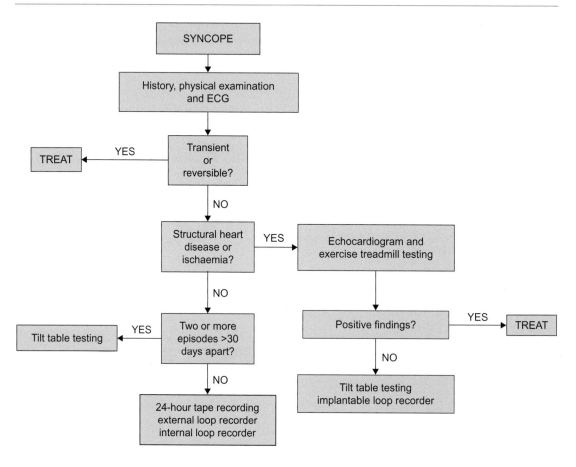

Adapted from Zimetbaum P, *et al. Ann Intern Med* 1999;**130:**848–56.

3 INVESTIGATIONS

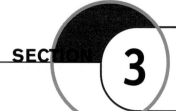

1. Decide whether the following statements are true or false

    a. Potassium requires urgent attention when between 4.0 and 6.5 mmol/L
    b. Magnesium concentrations tend to follow the trend of serum potassium concentrations
    c. There is a correlated rise in B-type natriuretic peptide levels as heart failure is successfully treated
    d. The D-dimer laboratory test is reliant on the non plasmin-mediated degradation of cross-linked fibrin clots

2. Concerning the D-dimer test and its use as a marker of DVT. Select the most appropriate response from the options provided

    a. It has a high specificity
    b. It has a high negative predictive value
    c. It has a low sensitivity
    d. It has a high positive predictive value
    e. It has poor accuracy

3. True or false? Troponin levels may be expected to rise in the following

    a. Myocardial infarction
    b. Pulmonary embolism
    c. Chronic renal failure
    d. A patient who has been lying on the floor for several hours after a collapse
    e. After a head injury

4. Which of the following are features of (i) troponin, (ii) CK or (iii) both?

    a. Cardio-specific
    b. Rises 4 hours post-myocardial infarction
    c. Persists for up to two weeks post-myocardial infarction
    d. In the context of myocardial infarction, the greater the rise, the larger the infarct
    e. Is expected to rise after significant skeletal damage

5. Concerning coronary disease, to what degree should total and LDL cholesterol levels be lowered?

CK, creatine kinase

EXPLANATION: CARDIAC-RELATED BLOOD TESTS

Full blood count

- Anaemia: should be **corrected in any patient with angina or breathlessness**
- White cell count: raised in inflammation (e.g. **pericarditis**) and infection (e.g. **endocarditis**, **rheumatic fever**).

Electrolytes and important markers

- Potassium: normal between 3.5 and 5.0 mmol/L; immediate action is required if below 2.5 or above 6.7
- Magnesium: normal range 0.7–1.1 mmol/L; magnesium tends to **follow the trend of potassium** (i.e. high when potassium is high)
- B-type natriuretic peptide: a test for heart failure; normally it is present in the blood at low levels, but **failing heart muscle secretes additional amounts; with successful treatment of the condition, there is a reduction in circulating levels**
- D-dimer: this is an end product derived from plasmin-mediated degradation of cross-linked fibrin clots; **high negative predictive value** for DVT and pulmonary embolism (i.e. low D-dimer = low probability of either condition).

Cardiac biomarkers

Damage to the myocardium causes the release of cardiac molecules (biomarkers). These are particularly useful in the context of chest pain, which may be the result of infarction. Biomarker results are used to diagnose MI in the context of clinical and ECG findings.

- Troponins: troponin T and troponin I are equally sensitive, though the latter is more specific; a more **cardio-specific** indicator of myocardial damage than older markers such as CK; begins to **rise 4 hours post-MI, peaking at around 12–24 hours** and remaining **raised for up to two weeks;** infarction is diagnosed when there is a rise above the upper normal limit; concentration can also quantify the **degree of injury** and hence the risk of complications; not entirely specific, as there are other common causes of raised troponin, including **pulmonary embolus**, **chronic renal failure** and **infection**
- CK: An older marker that is much less cardio-specific than troponin, as it can also rise after damage to skeletal muscle and brain tissue; levels **peak at 24 hours post-MI** and **fall within 36–48 hours**
- Cholesterol/triglycerides: lower total and LDL cholesterol confer reduced risk of development or progression of coronary disease; the degree to which lipid levels should be lowered by treatment is debated perennially (since there are diminishing returns for progressively stronger treatment); individual countries set guidelines such as '5 mmol/L total cholesterol and 3 mmol/L LDL cholesterol' for moderate-risk populations, or '4 mmol/L total cholesterol and 2 mmol/L LDL cholesterol' for high-risk populations such as those who have required coronary intervention **(5)**.

Answers

1. F T F F
2. b
3. T T T F F
4. (i) a, b, c; (ii) e; (iii) d
5. See explanation

A 55-year-old barman has a two-week history of chest pain on exertion. The pain is not associated with diaphoresis, shortness of breath, nausea or palpitations. Over the last week, he has been seen in an A&E department on two separate occasions. Cardiac enzymes/troponin T, chest radiography and ECG have not shown any abnormalities. He denies illicit drug use, but admits to having smoked 20 cigarettes per day for at least 30 years. He has been asked to carry out an ETT.

---

6. What is the purpose of an ETT?

---

7. Why, at this stage, is the test a suitable investigation for this man's symptoms?

---

8. Which ONE of the following is the most reliable indicator of exercise-induced ischaemia, in the context of this test?

    a. 1 mm of upsloping ST depression at a moderate workload
    b. 0.5 mm of downsloping ST depression at a minimal workload
    c. 1 mm of horizontal ST depression at a minimal workload
    d. 2 mm of upsloping ST depression at a minimal workload
    e. Chest pain induced at a minimal workload

---

9. Which of the following is NOT routinely monitored during the test (true or false)?

    a. Pulse   **d.** Pulse oximetry
    b. Blood pressure   **e.** Dizziness
    c. Chest pain

---

10. The man gives a positive test. Which of the following may also cause a positive ETT result in the absence of underlying disease (i.e. false positive) (true or false)?

    a. Left ventricular outflow obstruction   **d.** Fluoxetine
    b. Syndrome X   **e.** Varicose veins
    c. Imipramine

ETT, exercise treadmill test; HOCM, hypertrophic obstructive cardiomyopathy

EXPLANATION: EXERCISE TREADMILL TESTING

At rest, **coronary artery disease** generally manifests with minimal symptoms and unremarkable ECG changes. ETT aims to unmask underlying disease by exposing the heart to increasing levels of exercise. Under such conditions, healthy coronary vessels are able to dilate and increase blood flow to the myocardium, but narrow, diseased vessels maintain a reduced blood supply, increasing the likelihood of both ischaemic symptoms (e.g. chest pain) and ischaemic ECG changes (ST depression). The intensity and duration of the test is determined by a chosen protocol; the **Bruce protocol** is the most popular. Continuous **12-lead ECG**, **BP** and **pulse** monitoring are undertaken. The test is terminated if the patient desires, if the patient is at risk, when the criteria have been met for a positive test or when the test is completed (rare). The most widely examined ECG indicator of exercise-induced ischaemia is **ST segment depression**. To be significant, it should be at least **1 mm below the baseline and either horizontal or downsloping**.

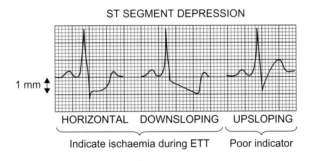

Essentially, ETT is a means of assessing the probability of ischaemic heart disease. In doing so, it enables us to identify patients who fall into the low-risk group for whom further investigation is not required. If the test is positive, the patient may undergo coronary angiography, which is a more accurate measure of coronary artery disease.

The false-positive rate increases with age, with a range of 5–20 per cent. The sensitivity of the test is in the region of 75 per cent (i.e. this is the prevalence of positive tests in a population who truly have coronary artery disease). Morbidity and mortality are relatively low: 24 and 10 in 100 000, respectively.

Possible causes of a false-positive test result	Features of ETT that warrant angiography	Contraindications to ETT
Cardiomyopathy	ST depression at low workload	Acute MI (within 5 days of test)
Hypertension	Failure of blood pressure to rise during exercise	Severe aortic stenosis
HOCM	Ventricular arrhythmias	Acute pulmonary embolism
Aortic stenosis		
Hyperventilation		
Syndrome X		
Electrolyte abnormalities		
Tricyclic antidepressant drugs		

Answers

6. To assess the *probability* of ischaemic heart disease
7. History of chest pain on exertion with normal resting ECG, background of cardiovascular risk factors (male, smoker)
8. c
9. d
10. T T T (tricyclic antidepressant) F (SSRI antidepressant) F

11. A 54-year-old man has been suffering with chest pain on exertion for almost 1
    year. After a recent ETT, which was highly positive, he was diagnosed with angina
    and started on a range of anti-anginal medications. In view of the ETT result, he has
    been asked to see you in an outpatient clinic. On reading his last clinic letter, you
    note that he also has chronic renal failure and osteoarthritis. An echocardiogram
    report shows normal LV function

   a. What is the most important question you should ask this patient to assess his current
      condition?
   b. In light of the strongly positive exercise treadmill test result, what would you suggest as
      the next appropriate investigative technique?
   c. How does this technique differ when visualizing the right rather than the left side of the
      heart?

12. The patient agrees to the investigation and is placed on the list for the next day.
    During the investigation, it is noted that he has severe single-vessel disease

   a. When choosing between percutaneous coronary intervention and coronary artery
      bypass grafting, which one is the most appropriate based on this result?
   b. What else in this man's history would steer you towards using one of these treatment
      strategies over the other?

13. State true or false for each of the following statements

   a. Subsequent coronary artery bypass grafting in a person who has previously undergone
      the procedure carries an increased risk of mortality
   b. The risk of myocardial infarction associated with coronary artery bypass grafting is
      decreased in the presence of peripheral vascular disease
   c. 'Plain old balloon angioplasty' leads to restenosis in 80 per cent of patients within six
      months
   d. Percutaneous stenting carries a higher risk of restenosis compared with 'plain old
      balloon angioplasty'
   e. For several weeks post-stenting, thrombus formation is prevented by administration of
      aspirin or clopidogrel

ETT, exercise treadmill test; PCI, percutaneous coronary intervention; POBA, 'plain old balloon angiography'

EXPLANATION: CARDIAC CATHETERIZATION

Cardiac catheterization is an **invasive technique** used to obtain detailed information about cardiac lesions or abnormalities when non-invasive techniques (e.g. ETT) have failed to do so or have merely suggested the presence of an underlying pathology. It is a dynamic technique that can also be used to treat some of the irregularities that it locates. The right side of the heart is accessed via one of the great veins (e.g. femoral vein), while the left side requires a peripheral artery (e.g. femoral artery); a catheter is then guided into the area being studied. **Coronary angiography** is the injection of radiopaque contrast (monitored by radiography) via the catheter. It provides a means of imaging the coronary anatomy and determining any impedance to blood flow. In coronary artery disease, one of two treatment strategies may be employed to bring about revascularization.

PCI: An angioplasty catheter is inserted into a coronary artery and a balloon is inflated at the site of an obstructing atheroma, thereby dilating the lumen. In most cases, a metal stent (cylindrical wire-mesh tube) is inflated into position at the site of the lesion. It is the first-choice therapy for most patients with one-, two- or three-vessel disease. The principal problem with angioplasty is restenosis, typically within six months. In angioplasty without stenting (nicknamed '**POBA**') restenosis occurs in about one-third of cases. Stenting has reduced this rate to around 10 per cent, and use of drug-eluting stents has further reduced it to 1–2 per cent. To prevent **thrombosis**, for the first few weeks after the procedure (while the endothelium has not yet grown over the stent) a combination of **aspirin** and **clopidogrel** must be given.

CABG: For almost all patients, this is a riskier procedure than PCI, because the chest has to be opened and the patient must be ventilated. Stopping the heart (cardiopulmonary bypass) also carries risks, but in many cases the procedure can be done on a beating heart ('off-pump' CABG). Serious complications (e.g. death/MI/wound infection) are increased with:

- Age
- Chronic renal failure
- Previous CABG
- Peripheral vascular disease
- Diastolic murmur
- Triple-vessel disease
- Impaired LV function.

The prognostic effect of these interventions on modern patients with stable symptoms is hard to evaluate, because the few randomized controlled trials were done decades ago when background medical therapy was very weak (e.g. no routine statin use). There is no doubt that both PCI and CABG are highly effective at alleviating symptoms. In acute coronary syndrome, these interventions have also been shown to improve prognosis, even on a background of modern medical therapy.

Stenting with a balloon catheter

1. A balloon catheter, carrying a stent, is usually passed into a vessel in the groin and fed up a coronary vessel

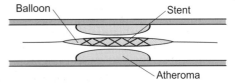

2. The ballon is inflated and the wire mesh stent expands, compressing the artheroma. There is a reduction in the stenosis

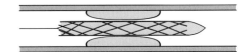

3. The stent is left behind, as the balloon is deflated and removed. It will be incorporated into the endothelial wall within several weeks

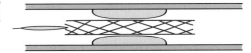

Answers

11. a – A suitable question about his chest pain since he started anti-anginals, b – Coronary angiography, c – Artery for left, vein for right
12. a – PCI, b – Chronic renal failure increases risk of serious complications in CABG
13. T F F F F

14. **Match the correct echocardiographic technique given below with the following statements. You may use the same option more than once**

Options

    A. Transoesophageal echocardiography
    B. Colour Doppler
    C. 2-Dimensional echocardiography
    D. M-mode echocardiography
    E. Doppler echocardiography

    1. Creates images that are interpreted with a simultaneous electrocardiogram recording
    2. Of all of the techniques, this has the highest sensitivity for the detection of cardiac vegetations that are the result of infective endocarditis
    3. This technique would be most suitable for the assessment of valvular regurgitation
    4. Almost always used to gather reference images for some of the other echocardiographic techniques
    5. This technique uses the direction and velocity of blood flow to evaluate cardiovascular haemodynamics

15. **The image below was obtained by 2-D echocardiography. Label the four major chambers of the heart on the image**

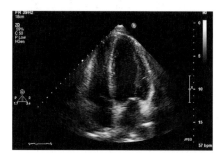

TOE, transoesophageal echocardiography

EXPLANATION: ECHOCARDIOGRAPHY

Echocardiograpy is a **non-invasive** technique in which high-pitched sound waves are reflected off the heart and then summarized in pictorial form. Interpretation of these images allows functional and anatomical assessment of cardiac structures. With the exception of TOE, images are acquired through the anterior chest wall (transthoracic approach). Echocardiography is considered the imaging technique of choice when evaluating **valvular disease**.

2-D ECHOCARDIOGRAPHY
Only after first gaining a reference from 2-D echocardiography would one go on to obtain M-mode and Doppler echocardiograms. In its own right, the technique is preferred when assessing **valve morphology** and **LV function**. By transmitting ultrasound beams at a **series of angles**, this imaging technique obtains data that are used to create a **cross-sectional image of the heart**. This image represents a slice of the heart at its intersection with the imaging plane.

M-MODE
This is generally used to detail accurate measurements of **individual heart structures**. Data are collected from a single ultrasound beam over time. The picture formed is interpreted with the aid of a simultaneous ECG recording.

DOPPLER ECHOCARDIOGRAPHY
Doppler echocardiography uses the principle of **Doppler shift** to gather information regarding the **flow of blood** within the heart and its vessels. Colour Doppler takes this a step further, by assigning a value to each pixel in the image corresponding to both **the direction and the magnitude of the blood velocity**. By convention, blood flowing towards the imaging device is denoted by the colour **red** and that flowing away by the colour **blue**, with **green** indicating turbulent flow (e.g. across a valve).

TOE
The chest wall and lungs impede ultrasound beams directed towards the heart. In TOE, **the imaging probe is placed down the patient's oesophagus**, resulting in higher-resolution images with greater structural clarity. TOE is favoured in situations where transthoracic techniques are technically difficult (e.g. during surgery). It also has special value in imaging areas that are not well visualized by transthoracic imaging (e.g. the interatrial septum, parts of the aorta when looking for an aortic dissection) or when examining an already abnormal aortic or mitral valve for evidence of vegetation. Metal prosthetic valves create a large acoustic shadow, so that the 'far' side of the valve cannot be seen well. Combining transthoracic and transoesophageal imaging in such a patient allows imaging of the whole heart. TOE is also used in cases involving prosthetic valves or congenital abnormalities and in patients with systemic emboli in whom a cardiac defect is suspected but cannot be identified by standard transthoracic techniques.

16. Concerning stress echocardiography (true or false?)

a. It is the next line of investigation when a patient is unable to perform an exercise treadmill test
b. Adenosine is given to reproduce physiological stress on the heart
c. The heart is imaged during the stress component of the procedure
d. It is contraindicated if there is a history of myocardial infarction
e. It is contraindicated if there is a history of diastolic murmur

17. Concerning myocardial perfusion imaging (true or false?)

a. It assesses myocardial blood flow
b. It assesses myocyte integrity
c. Technetium-99 binds irreversibly to the surface of myocytes
d. Images are gathered by a gamma camera
e. It can determine prognosis for patients with acute myocardial infarction

18. Concerning PET of the heart (true or false?)

a. Hypoperfused myocytes revert from glycolytic to fatty acid metabolism
b. It uses fluorine-18-labelled glucose tracer agent to penetrate myocytes
c. If PET is inconclusive, coronary angiography is typically the next line of investigation
d. It is the next line of investigation when the results of myocardial perfusion scanning are inconclusive
e. It uses dipyridamole to induce myocardial ischaemia

19. Concerning CT

a. It is the modality of choice when investigating the ascending component of the aorta
b. It is the modality of choice when investigating the descending component of the aorta
c. It is the diagnostic gold standard for dissecting aortic aneurysm
d. It is typically used in the assessment of constrictive pericarditis
e. It uses iodine-based contrast agents

20. Concerning cardic MRI

a. High-resolution gated images are possible
b. It may be used to assess perfusion defects
c. Gadolinium contrast is used to assess viable and non-viable myocardial tissue
d. It is unsuitable for patients with implanted pacemakers
e. It is suitable for imaging valvular heart defects

PET, positron emission tomography; ETT, exercise treadmill test

EXPLANATION: ADDITIONAL CARDIAC SCANS

Stress echocardiography: This is generally reserved for patients who are unable to perform an ETT, typically due to poor mobility. Stressing agents (e.g. dobutamine, arbutamine) are given with the intention of reproducing the heart's physiological response to exercise. This is beneficial, as echocardiography can be used during the 'stress' session to capture the characteristically weak contraction of ischaemic myocardium. Furthermore, atropine and dipyridamole can be used to augment the heart's response to the pharmaceutical stress.

Myocardial perfusion imaging: This assesses regional myocardial blood flow and the integrity of myocytes, with the patient at rest and then after exercise. An injected radiolabelled agent (e.g. thallium-201, technetium-99) is distributed through the myocardium via the coronary vessels. The agent then crosses the cellular membranes of functioning myocytes and remains irreversibly trapped within the cells, but visible to a gamma camera. The quantity of agent correlates well with the degree of perfusion, areas of infarction (fixed defects) showing little or none. To establish the presence of ischaemic zones (reversible defects), the heart is visualized after strenuous exercise; agent levels are initially low and reach normal values as the patient recovers. The technique is useful in the diagnosis of coronary artery disease and is increasingly used to evaluate the prognosis following acute MI.

PET: In severely hypoperfused myocytes, metabolic processes change from fatty acid to glycolytic. Approximately 40 per cent of thallium-201 scans visualize these areas as fixed defects when they actually contain tissue that is functionally viable in the presence of normal blood flow. When patients are injected with fluorine-18-labelled deoxyglucose, it is utilized at these sites and can be imaged by PET. PET is generally used to gather further information when the results of myocardial perfusion imaging or coronary angiography are inconclusive.

CT: This is the modality of choice when assessing the descending and ascending components of the aorta. Although MRI is the gold standard for diagnosing a dissecting aortic aneurysm, CT is the preferred imaging technique as it is comparatively cheaper. CT provides limited images of intracardiac structures, with the exception of the atria and the pericardial space (e.g. constrictive pericarditis). Iodine-based contrast agents are used to opacify blood within the heart, so that structural abnormalities are more identifiable.

Cardiac MRI: This is an established imaging tool for intracardiac structures, congenital heart defects, cardiac masses and the great vessels. Unlike CT, it can produce high-resolution gated images (i.e. still images at any point during the cardiac cycle), with the added benefit of not exposing the patient to radiation. The addition of gadolinium contrast is a relatively new technique that allows assessment of viable and non-viable myocardial tissue post-MI. The technique is also being used to assess perfusion defects during acute MI.

Answers

16. T F T F F
17. T T F T T
18. F F F T F
19. T T F T T
20. T T T T T

SECTION 4

THE ELECTROCARDIOGRAM

1. Label the diagram below to show where you would place the chest leads to obtain an ECG

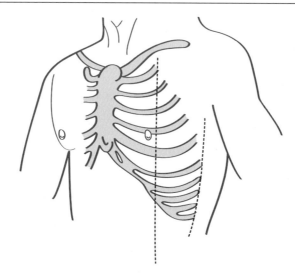

2. Name the important bony landmark that allows correct positioning of the precordial leads

3. For each chest lead, describe which aspect of the heart it looks at

4. Describe Einthoven's triangle and how it is used to view the heart's vertical plane

5. In the UK, specific colours are used to represent ECG limb leads. Using the options provided, match each of the limb leads with its correct colour

Options

A. Right shoulder
B. Left shoulder
C. Upper part of left thigh
D. Upper part of right thigh

1. Red
2. Blue
3. Yellow
4. Green
5. Brown
6. Grey
7. Orange
8. Purple
9. Black

ICS, intercostal space

EXPLANATION: RECORDING AN ELECTROCARDIOGRAM

An **electrocardiograph** is an instrument used to measure the intrinsic electrical impulses of the heart via electrodes placed on the body surface. The recording is an **electrocardiogram**, which represents the activity as a series of oscillations. Oscillations from a normal cardiac cycle are named **P**, **Q**, **R**, **S** and **T** and follow in alphabetical order. Additional letters may be necessary for other distinct waveforms. 12-Lead ECG uses ten physical electrodes placed on the patient. A lead looks at a particular aspect of the heart and may be either unipolar (**V1–V6**, **aVR**, **aVL** and **aVF**) or bipolar (**I**, **II** and **III**).

SIX PRECORDIAL LEADS (CHEST LEADS)
These are six unipolar leads that provide a view of the heart's horizontal plane **(1)**.

Lead	Placement	Aspect of the heart (3)
V1	Fourth ICS right sternal edge	RV
V2	Fourth ICS left sternal edge	
V3	Half-way between V2 and V4	Ventricular septum and anterior wall of the LV
V4	Mid-clavicular line, fifth ICS over apex	
V5	Same level as V4 on anterior axillary line	Anterior and lateral walls of the LV
V6	Same level as V4 on mid-axillary line	

The sternal angle **(2)** is a bony landmark frequently used to locate the second ICS. Slide your fingers a little to the right and they should fall into this dip; passing your fingers inferiorly and over two ribs takes you into the fourth ICS, the location for V1 and the reference point for V2.

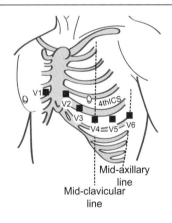

SIX LIMB LEADS
In the UK, the four electrodes used are: red – right shoulder, yellow – left shoulder, green – upper part of left thigh, and black – upper part of right thigh (colours vary in the USA). Importantly, the information from these electrodes (bar the black electrode, which is neutral) is combined to form Einthoven's triangle **(4)** (shown below), creating six limb lead views across the heart's vertical plane.

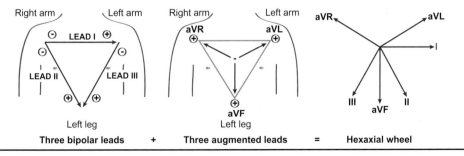

Answers
1. See diagram
2. Sternal angle. See explanation
3. See explanation
4. See explanation
5. 1 – A, 3 – B, 4 – C, 9 – D

6. Using leads aVR and II, describe the effect of electrical movement on the ECG tracings of two leads viewing the heart from opposite directions

7. What is the standard speed for ECG tracings?

8. Describe the paper used for ECG tracings. What do the squares represent?

9. What is a calibration signal?

EXPLANATION: LEADS AND PAPER

The **hexaxial wheel** depicts each limb lead as an imaginary line between a negative pole (the centre of the hexaxial wheel) and a positive pole (a point towards the periphery of the wheel). Electrical activity is said to be moving towards a particular lead when it travels from the negative to the positive pole, which is seen as an **upward deflection** in the lead on the final ECG tracing. You can therefore appreciate that if electrical activity is travelling away from the lead (i.e. from the positive to the negative pole), this will cause a **downward deflection** in the respective lead.

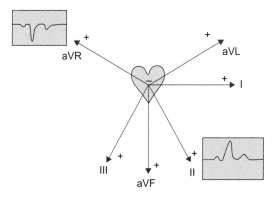

As leads aVR and II record electrical activity from opposite directions (approximately) their respective tracings are mirror reflections across the horizontal axis (6)

12-Lead ECG is an attempt to create a sphere of 12 recording views around the heart, each observing overall electrical activity. It is possible to use the ECG to calculate not only the direction of electrical activity (using **vectors**), but also to determine the presence of certain cardiac pathologies that give characteristically abnormal tracings.

ECG paper moves through the machine at a standard speed of **25 mm/second (7)**. The paper comprises **small 1 mm squares** and **large 5 mm squares**. Each small square represents **0.04 seconds (one large square = 0.2 seconds) (8)**. A **calibration signal** or spike should always be shown on an ECG tracing; it is generally one large square across (informing the reader that the machine is set to the standard 25 mm/second) and two large squares in height (which represents **1 mV) (9)**.

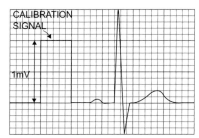

Answers

6. See explanation
7. See explanation
8. See explanation
9. See explanation

10. Match each of the following statements with the correct options provided on the diagram below. You may use the same answer more than once or not at all

Options

1. Generally inverted when ischaemic changes are present
2. Represents 0.2 seconds
3. Absence suggests atrial fibrillation
4. Indicative of hypercalcaemia and hyperkalaemia
5. Represents 1 mV
6. Represents septal activation

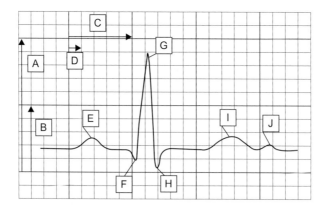

11. True or false? The following characteristically result in bradycardia

a. Hypothermia
b. Angiotensin-converting enzyme inhibitors
c. Structural sinoatrial node disease
d. Atropine
e. Anaemia

12. True or false? The following characteristically result in tachycardia

a. Thyrotoxicosis
b. Obstructive jaundice
c. Hypovolaemia
d. Myocarditis
e. Adrenergic blockade

EXPLANATION: BASIC ELECTROCARDIOGRAM INTERPRETATION (I)

Outlined below are the important components that may exist on an ECG tracing; some of them may not always be present and this may be the result of pathology or a normal ECG. (NB: The terms **upward** and **downward deflection** are relative to the baseline that exists before the P wave.)

P wave: Height should be 2.5 small squares and width 2–3 small squares. This represents atrial depolarization and is the first upward deflection on a tracing. Such waves may be tall in right atrial hypertrophy, wide in left atrial hypertrophy or inverted in dextrocardia. In atrial fibrillation, normal depolarization is not possible, as the atria are bombarded by a storm of electrical impulses and the ECG shows an absence of P waves.

QRS complex: Width should be less than 3 small squares. As a whole, the QRS complex signifies ventricular depolarization. Complexes may be small, as may be seen in obesity, emphysema and pericardial effusion. Widening of the complex is usually observed in patients with bundle branch block (see pages 51 and 53).

Q wave: This is the first downward deflection of the QRS complex and represents early septal activation. Small Q waves, called q waves, may be seen in normal subjects in the first few chest leads (V1 and V2). Deep and wide Q waves are always pathological.

R wave: Height should be less than 25 small squares in V5 or V6. It is the result of ventricular depolarization spreading through the ventricles, forcing an upward deflection in the QRS complex. 'R wave progression' refers to the lack of (in V1) and the subsequent increase in the height of the R wave (from lead V2 up to V5).

S wave: Depth should be less than 25 small squares in V1 or V2. This is the downward deflection immediately after an R wave (therefore no R wave present = no S wave present). The wave is normally deepest in V1 and decreases in size to V5–V6, where it may be absent.

T wave: The result of ventricular repolarization, this is a relatively small upward bump just after a QRS complex. It is normally inverted in the aVR lead and upright in I, II and V3–V6. Tall T waves are associated with severe hyperkalaemia (tented T waves) or very early MI. Abnormally inverted T waves may be seen in ischaemia, infarction, ventricular hypertrophy, bundle branch block and cerebral disease.

U wave: Seen best in V2–V4. This is an upward bump immediately after a T wave. Its presence is indicative of hypokalaemia and hypercalcaemia.

Answers
10. 1 – I, 2 – C, 3 – E, 4 – J, 5 – A, 6 – F
11. T F T F F
12. T F T T F

13. Lengthening of the PR interval indicates some form of heart block. Which one the following statements is the most suitable answer? The normal duration for a PR interval is

a. 0.12–0.2 seconds
b. 1.2–2.0 seconds
c. 0.15–0.2 seconds
d. 0.2–0.4 seconds
e. 0.1–0.12 seconds

14. Concerning the QRS complex. Which of the following does NOT characteristically cause an increase in the duration of a QRS complex?

a. Incomplete left bundle branch block
b. Incomplete right bundle branch block
c. Non-specific intraventricular conduction delay
d. Anterior fascicular block
e. Second-degree heart block

15. Concerning the finding of ST depression. Match each of the options below with the voltage diagram most likely to be seen

Options

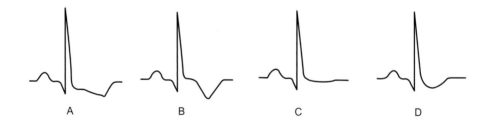

A   B   C   D

1. Non-specific abnormality
2. Digitalis effect
3. Strain as a result of right ventricular hypertrophy
4. Strain as a result of left ventricular hypertrophy

EXPLANATION: BASIC ELECTROCARDIOGRAM INTERPRETATION (II)

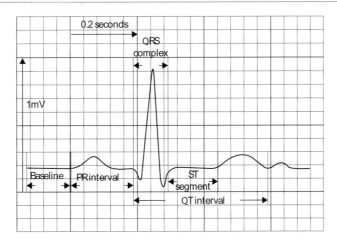

PR interval: Normally 3–5 small squares (0.12–0.2 seconds). This is measured from the beginning of atrial depolarization to the beginning of ventricular depolarization. A prolonged interval corresponds with impaired atrioventricular node conduction and indicates heart block (see page 45).

QRS complex: Normally less than 2.5 small squares (0.1 seconds). Lengthening implies conduction delay through the ventricles.

ST segment: This is the part of the tracing that lies between the end of the QRS complex and the beginning of the T wave. It should be fairly even with the baseline. Depression below or elevation above the baseline may indicate myocardial ischaemia or MI, respectively (see pages 73 and 79).

QT interval: The QT interval may be prolonged by electrolyte abnormalities such as hypokalaemia, hypocalcaemia and hypomagnesaemia, or by myocardial ischaemia. It is a measure of the time between the start of the Q wave and the end of the T wave. At normal heart rates, the QT length is abnormal if it is greater than 10 small squares (0.40 seconds) in males and 11 small squares (0.44 seconds) in females. Extreme QT prolongation (>15 small squares, 0.60 seconds) predisposes the patient to arrhythmias.

Corrected QT (QTc) interval: This is measured in a somewhat unintuitive way, from the beginning of the QRS to the end of the T wave. Because it varies with heart rate, it is 'corrected' by dividing by the RR interval in seconds. So, when the heart rate is 60 bpm, the QTc is simply the QT interval. When the heart rate is 30 bpm, the RR interval is 2 seconds, so the QTc is $QT/\sqrt{2}$. The upper limit for the QTc is 460 ms in men and 470 ms in women.

Answers

13. a

14. e

15. A – 4 (asymmetrical ST depression), B – 3 (symmetrical ST depression), C – 1, D – 2 (digoxin may cause a 'scooping' effect as in the diagram, a strain pattern or no change)

16. A hexaxial wheel (axis wheel) is drawn below. It shows how the six limb leads monitor the same cardiac electrical activity, from six different angles. Match the lead options provided to their corresponding angle of measurement

Options

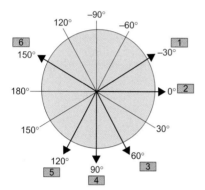

A. Lead III
B. aVL
C. aVF
D. Lead I
E. aVR
F. Lead II

17. The hexaxial wheel has also been split into 12 sectors. Shade the sectors that represent

a. Right axis deviation   c. Normal axis
b. Left axis deviation

18. The conditions below are commonly associated with either (1) right axis deviation or (2) left axis deviation. Match the options correctly

a. Dextrocardia
b. Right ventricular hypertrophy
c. Severe chronic obstructive airway disease
d. Left anterior fascicular block

f. Left ventricular hypertrophy
g. Lateral wall myocardial infarction
h. Inferior wall
e. Left posterior fascicular block

19. Five separate ECG tracings are tabulated below. Using the information provided, determine the axis deviation in each subject

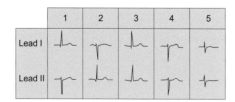

EXPLANATION: RATE AND AXIS

RATE

One of two methods may be used to calculate heart rate (ventricular rate), depending on whether the rhythm strip is regular or irregular.

Regular rhythm: Divide 300 by the number of large squares separating the R wave in one QRS complex and the R wave of the subsequent QRS complex (RR interval).

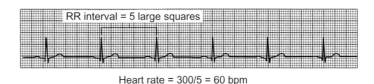

Heart rate = 300/5 = 60 bpm

Irregular rhythm: Calculate the number of QRS complexes within 30 large squares and multiply by 10.

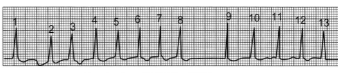

Heart rate = 13 X 10 = 130 bpm

Asynchronous contraction between the atria and ventricles (e.g. third-degree block) requires use of the PP interval in addition to the ventricular techniques shown above. You will then have both the atrial and the ventricular rates.

AXIS

The 'axis' of an ECG generally refers to the **mean frontal plane QRS axis**. A 'normal axis' is taken to be between 0 and 90°, where 0 is the easterly line on the hexaxial wheel. Deviation from the normal range is a fairly blunt-edged tool for diagnostic purposes, but it may provide evidence on the source of any ECG abnormalities (e.g. right axis deviation suggests right-sided heart disease, left axis deviation can feature with inferior MI). Using the positive or negative deflections of the QRS complex in both leads I and II gives a quick and simple method for approximating the axis (see diagram).

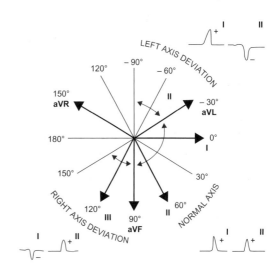

Answers

16. A – 5, B – 1, C – 4, D – 2, E – 6, F – 3
17. Fig. 4.14 (right)
18. (1) b, e, g, (2) a, c, d, f, h
19. 1 – left axis deviation, 2 – right axis deviation, 3 – normal axis, 4 – superior right axis deviation (+150° to +270°), 5 – indeterminate axis (isoelectric in lead I and II)

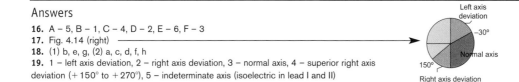

20. Describe the anatomical location of the AV node and outline the node's function in pathological circumstances

21. Case study. The ECG tracing below was taken from a 45-year-old man who was seen by his GP for a routine check-up. Name and describe the abnormality shown

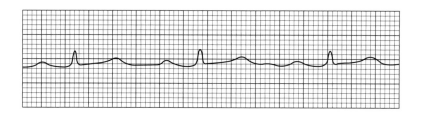

22. Which of the following may cause this condition? (true or false)

    a. Enhanced vagal tone
    b. Acute myocardial infarction
    c. Electrolyte disturbances
    d. Atenolol
    e. Calcium channel blockers

23. No other abnormalities were seen on the ECG. For the management of this patient (true or false)

    a. He should undergo repeat electrocardiography after two weeks to ensure that the abnormality has resolved
    b. He requires urgent referral to a cardiologist
    c. Any electrolyte disturbances found on blood tests should be corrected
    d. He should be informed that the prognosis associated with this abnormality is relatively good
    e. He should inform the DVLA, as he will not be allowed to drive until his condition has resolved

AV, atrioventricular; SA, sinoatrial

EXPLANATION: FIRST-DEGREE ATRIOVENTRICULAR BLOCK

Normally, waves of depolarization spread through the heart's internal conduction system in the following manner: **SA node (atria)** → **AV node (beginning of ventricles)** → **His bundle (middle of ventricles)** → **bundle branches (middle of ventricles)** → **Purkinje fibres**. All parts of the conduction system, as well as the myocardial cells (myocytes), are capable of initiating impulses to start a cardiac cycle.

AV node: The AV node provides a pathway of minimal resistance for impulses coming from the SA node; it is located on the **interatrial septum**, close to the tricuspid valve **(20)**. Normally, impulses are delayed within the AV node, ensuring that the ventricles are given sufficient filling time before they contract. This can be protective in pathological circumstances such as atrial fibrillation, where the AV node may receive up to 300 impulses per minute, transmitting only a small proportion of these to the ventricles **(20)**. Furthermore, the His bundle and AV node form AV junctional tissue. This has intrinsic pacemaker activity (in the region of 40–60 bpm), allowing it to take over the heart's rhythm when the functioning of the SA node is impaired.

The time it takes for an impulse to travel from the atria to the ventricles (the **PR interval**) should be less than 0.2 seconds (5 small squares); any longer than this is termed first-degree AV block. In such cases, impulses from the atria are consistently delayed as they pass through the AV node, but eventually get through. Electrophysiological studies have shown that first-degree block may be due to conduction delay in the AV node, in the His-Purkinje system, or in a combination of the two. It is generally an **incidental finding** noted on ECG with no clinically apparent signs.

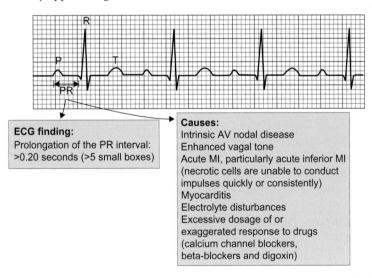

ECG finding:
Prolongation of the PR interval: >0.20 seconds (>5 small boxes)

Causes:
Intrinsic AV nodal disease
Enhanced vagal tone
Acute MI, particularly acute inferior MI (necrotic cells are unable to conduct impulses quickly or consistently)
Myocarditis
Electrolyte disturbances
Excessive dosage of or exaggerated response to drugs (calcium channel blockers, beta-blockers and digoxin)

First-degree AV block does not require hospital admission, unless it is associated with MI. Electrolyte abnormalities should be identified and corrected, and any offending medications removed from the patient's prescription. The prognosis of first-degree heart block is very good.

Answers
20. See explanation
21. First-degree AV block (PR interval >0.2 seconds)
22. T T T T T
23. F F T T F

24. The following rhythm strip is from lead II of an ECG tracing. Identify the correct rhythm, from the options provided

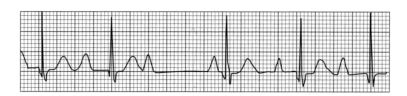

a. Normal sinus rhythm
b. First-degree atrioventricular block
c. Type I second-degree block

d. Type II second-degree block
e. Third-degree atrioventricular block

25. The following rhythm strip is from lead II of an ECG tracing. Identify the correct rhythm, from the options provided

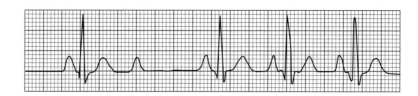

a. Normal sinus rhythm
b. First-degree atrioventricular block
c. Type I second-degree block

d. Type II second-degree block
e. Third-degree atrioventricular block

26. Concerning AV heart block (true or false?)

a. Patients with type I second-degree block are rarely asymptomatic
b. Patients with type II second-degree block should undergo cardiac monitoring before the correction of any reversible causes
c. Patients with type II second-degree block are normally given atropine to restore cardiac synchrony
d. Temporary pacing is contraindicated in patients with type II second-degree block who are experiencing dyspnoea
e. Patients with type II second-degree block may present with cardiovascular collapse

AV, atrioventricular

EXPLANATION: SECOND-DEGREE ATRIOVENTRICULAR BLOCK

Second-degree block can be of two types: **Mobitz I (Wenckebach)** and **Mobitz II**. In **Mobitz I** there is a progressive delay of impulse conduction at the AV node, until conduction is completely blocked and there is a loss of ventricular contraction (a dropped beat). In **Mobitz II**, the PR interval is normal, but there is a sudden failure in conduction and hence contraction.

Mobitz I block is caused by conduction delay in the AV node in 72 per cent of patients and by conduction delay in the His-Purkinje system in the remaining 28 per cent. A narrow QRS complex makes the site of delay even more likely to be the AV node. Mobitz I block with a wide QRS complex may be due to AV nodal or infranodal conduction delay. Electrophysiological studies have proved that **Mobitz II** block is due to an infranodal His-Purkinje system conduction delay. It is generally associated with a wide QRS complex, except in cases where the delay is localized within the bundle of His.

Second-degree block: Mobitz type I

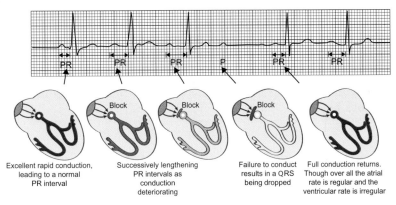

| Excellent rapid conduction, leading to a normal PR interval | Successively lengthening PR intervals as conduction deteriorating | Failure to conduct results in a QRS being dropped | Full conduction returns. Though over all the atrial rate is regular and the ventricular rate is irregular |

Second-degree block: Mobitz type II

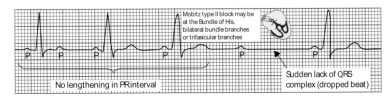

As **Mobitz I** block is usually **asymptomatic**, intervention is rarely required. In contrast, **Mobitz II** block carries a high risk of progression to **third-degree AV block** (a condition often associated with **cardiovascular collapse**). Patients should be closely monitored, paying particular attention to any reduction in cardiac output (e.g. tachycardia with subsequent hypotension). **Atropine**, **dopamine** or **epinephrine** may be used to treat symptomatic bradycardia. If reversible causes have been eliminated, patients generally undergo **temporary pacing** until a **permanent pacemaker** can be fitted.

Answers
24. c
25. d
26. F T F F T

27. Which of the following does not typically carry a risk of development of third-degree AV block?

a. Anterior wall myocardial infarction
b. Ventricular septal defect repair
c. Donepezil overdose
d. Propanolol
e. Captopril

28. With regard to third-degree AV block, is it true or false that

a. There is a 30 per cent reduction in the force of atrial contraction
b. Some of the QRS complexes observed on electrocardiography are initiated by the depolarization from P waves
c. Treatment aims to improve cardiac synchrony with a view to increasing cardiac output
d. The PR interval is expected to be less than 0.12 across the electrocardiogram rhythm strip
e. The ventricular rate is always slower than the atrial rate

29. The following rhythm strip is from lead II of an ECG tracing. Identify the correct rhythm, from the options provided

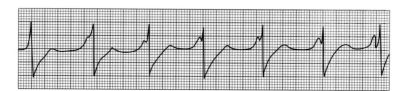

a. First-degree atrioventricular block
b. Type II second-degree block
c. 2:1 second-degree block
d. Third-degree atrioventricular block
e. Complete atrioventricular dissociation

AV, atrioventricular; SA, sinoatrial

EXPLANATION: THIRD-DEGREE ATRIOVENTRICULAR BLOCK (COMPLETE HEART BLOCK)

In third-degree AV block, impulses from the atria never reach the ventricles and the atria are no longer in synchrony with the ventricles. Instead, the ventricular rhythm is maintained by **pacemaker cells** that are associated with components lower down the conduction pathway. It is important to note that there is a tendency for the pacemaker cells to fire at a slower rate further down the system. Usually, the ventricular rhythm is maintained by pacemaker cells in the AV node (**junctional pacemaker**), resulting in narrow QRS complexes. In third-degree AV block localized to the bundle branches, the ventricular rhythm is maintained by a pacemaker in the Purkinje fibres, resulting in wide QRS complexes (i.e. a slower firing rate increases the duration of the QRS complex).

The rhythm observed on an ECG tracing has regular P waves that seem to be laid on top of a regular set of QRS complexes; sometimes P waves are buried within QRS complexes. The PR interval varies, some being greater and some less than 0.12 seconds (3 squares). Clinically, there is a 30 per cent reduction in blood transmitted from the atria to the ventricles, as they no longer contract in synchrony. Combine this with the slower rate of ventricular contraction (which may fall below 45 bpm) and you have a patient who is easily tipped into a state of haemodynamic compromise (e.g. on light exertion).

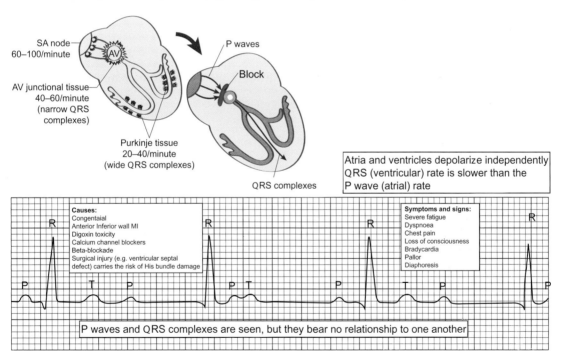

SA node
60–100/minute

P waves

Block

AV junctional tissue
40–60/minute
(narrow QRS
complexes)

Purkinje tissue
20–40/minute
(wide QRS complexes)

QRS complexes

Atria and ventricles depolarize independently
QRS (ventricular) rate is slower than the
P wave (atrial) rate

Causes:
Congentaial
Anterior Inferior wall MI
Digoxin toxicity
Calcium channel blockers
Beta-blockade
Surgical injury (e.g. ventricular septal
defect) carries the risk of His bundle damage

Symptoms and signs:
Severe fatigue
Dyspnoea
Chest pain
Loss of consciousness
Bradycardia
Pallor
Diaphoresis

P waves and QRS complexes are seen, but they bear no relationship to one another

Treatment aims to improve **cardiac synchrony** and hence cardiac output. **Atropine** may be used as a first-line anti-arrhythmic agent, but most patients are given temporary pacing until a permanent pacemaker can be fitted.

Answers

27. c (cholinesterase inhibitor used in Alzheimer's disease), e (ACE inhibitor)
28. F F T F T
29. e

30. RBBB is a common ECG finding. The schematic below shows a characteristic tracing that may be seen. Which lead should this be seen in to meet the diagnostic criteria for RBBB? Choose ONE answer from the options provided

a. V1
b. V4
c. III
d. aVR
e. I

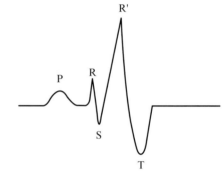

31. Following on from this, what are the other criteria that must be fulfilled so that a diagnosis of RBBB may be given?

32. True or false? The following significantly increase the risk of developing RBBB

a. Duchenne muscular dystrophy
b. *SCN5A* gene mutation
c. Atrial septal defect
d. Crohn's disease
e. Myotonic dystrophy

RBBB, right bundle branch block

EXPLANATION: RIGHT BUNDLE BRANCH BLOCK

As the name suggests, electrical impulses are prevented from travelling in the right bundle branch of the intraventricular conducting system (the His bundle). Instead, the RV must depolarize by slower cell-to-cell transmission, spreading from the interventricular septum and left bundle branch towards the right side of the heart. Incomplete RBBB is the development of the shape of RBBB without prolongation of the QRS width.

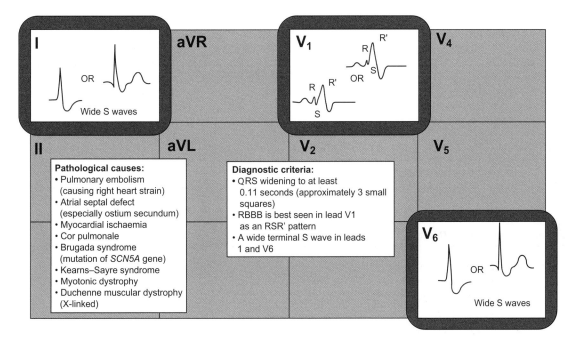

I

aVR

Wide S waves

II

aVL

Pathological causes:
• Pulmonary embolism
  (causing right heart strain)
• Atrial septal defect
  (especially ostium secundum)
• Myocardial ischaemia
• Cor pulmonale
• Brugada syndrome
  (mutation of *SCN5A* gene)
• Kearns–Sayre syndrome
• Myotonic dystrophy
• Duchenne muscular dystrophy
  (X-linked)

V_1

V_4

V_2

V_5

Diagnostic criteria:
• QRS widening to at least
  0.11 seconds (approximately 3 small
  squares)
• RBBB is best seen in lead V1
  as an RSR' pattern
• A wide terminal S wave in leads
  1 and V6

V_6

Wide S waves

Answers

30. a
31. See diagram
32. T T T F T

33. Which of the following statements concerning the ECG finding of LBBB is NOT true?

    a. Unlike right bundle branch block, it always indicates significant cardiac pathology
    b. It prevents any further interpretation of the ST segments on the electrocardiogram
    c. It is commonly the result of left ventricular dysfunction
    d. In the absence of contraindications, reperfusion therapy should be given (i.e. thrombolysis)
    e. The left ventricle of the heart depolarizes as impulses arrive from the right bundle branch and the interventricular septum

34. Which of the following are associated with an increased risk of developing LBBB (true or false)?

    a. Acromegaly
    b. Barth syndrome
    c. Cushing's syndrome
    d. Conn's syndrome
    e. Severe aortic stenosis

35. State the diagnostic criteria for LBBB

36. Explain, with the aid of a diagram, why complete RBBB is sometimes described as an 'M-shaped' pattern in lead V1. Why does this happen?

LBBB, left bundle branch block; RBBB, right bundle branch block

EXPLANATION: LEFT BUNDLE BRANCH BLOCK

Unlike RBBB, **LBBB always indicates significant cardiac pathology**, which is invariably due to **LV dysfunction**. Transmission of electrical impulses is prevented across the left bundle branch and they must instead travel from the interventricular septum and right bundle branch to the left side, through the myocardium. This transmission from the right to the left side of the septum is seen as a Q wave (downward) in V1 and a reciprocal R wave (upward) in V6. As the RV depolarizes first (as the LV is waiting to be initiated), there follows a small R wave in V1 with a reciprocal S wave in V6. Eventually, the LV depolarizes, creating a deep S wave in V1 and a tall R1 wave in V6. Globally, ST segments and T waves are abnormal, and this prevents any further interpretation of the ECG. For this reason, **patients with clinical features of myocardial ischaemia (e.g. chest pain) and new LBBB are presumed** to have had a MI until proven otherwise. Bar contraindications, they should be given reperfusion therapy (thrombolysis).

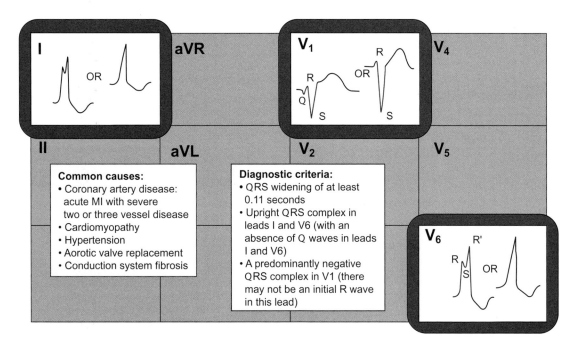

Common causes:
- Coronary artery disease: acute MI with severe two or three vessel disease
- Cardiomyopathy
- Hypertension
- Aortic valve replacement
- Conduction system fibrosis

Diagnostic criteria:
- QRS widening of at least 0.11 seconds
- Upright QRS complex in leads I and V6 (with an absence of Q waves in leads I and V6)
- A predominantly negative QRS complex in V1 (there may not be an initial R wave in this lead)

Morphology: The QRS complex in bundle branch block undergoes obvious morphological changes, and this can be explained by the ventricles depolarizing out of synchrony rather than in unison. Instead of a single wave, there are two R waves (R and R′) overlapping one another; the overlap accounts for the extended width of the complex and the characteristic 'M-shaped' morphology seen in V1 (RBBB) **(36)** and V6 (LBBB).

Continued on page 70

Answers

33. d
34. T (associated with coronary artery disease) T (causes dilated cardiomyopathy) T (associated with high BP) T (associated with high BP) F
35. See diagram
36. See explanation, continued on page 70

37. Match the following descriptions with the SINGLE most appropriate option from the list provided. Options may be used more than once or not at all

Options

A. Acute marginal branch
B. Left anterior descending artery
C. Septal branches
D. Obtuse marginal branches
E. Left circumflex artery
F. Left coronary artery

G. Right coronary artery
H. Diagonal branches
I. Posterior descending artery
J. Sinoatrial node
K. Atrioventricular node

1. This node receives its blood supply from both right and left coronary arteries
2. This node receives its blood supply solely from the right coronary artery
3. The artery that originates at the left coronary sinus
4. This artery travels within the left interventricular groove
5. Has obtuse marginal branches
6. In 85 per cent of the population, this is the dominant artery
7. Supplies the posteromedial papillary muscle
8. The artery that bifurcates into the left anterior descending artery and left circumflex artery

38. The vessel from which the posterior descending artery arises determines whether the coronary arteries exhibit left or right dominance or even co-dominance. Knowing this, together with your knowledge of the coronary arteries, which one of the following statements is correct?

a. In 70 per cent of the population, the right coronary artery is dominant
b. In 30 per cent of the population, the posterior descending artery arises from the circumflex artery
c. Co-dominance exists in 12–13 per cent of the population
d. The left circumflex artery supplies 15–25 per cent of the left ventricle in right-dominant systems
e. The posterior descending artery supplies the anterolateral papillary muscle in both right- and left-dominant systems

---

LCA, left coronary artery; RCA, right coronary artery; LAD, left anterior descending; LCx, left circumflex; AV, atrioventricular; SA, sinoatrial

EXPLANATION: ANATOMY AND TERRITORIES OF THE CORONARY ARTERIES (I)

Coronary vessels run across the surface of the heart and are capable of **autoregulation**, maintaining coronary flow at levels appropriate to the needs of the heart. Generally there are two main **coronary arteries**, the **left (LCA)** and **right (RCA)**. Both originate from their respective sinuses, superior to the left and right cusps of the aortic valve. It is important to note that the exact anatomy of the myocardial blood supply can vary considerably between individuals.

LCA: The LCA originates in the **left coronary sinus**. After a relatively short distance, it bifurcates into the **left anterior descending (LAD)** artery and the **left circumflex (LCx)** artery. In 37 per cent of the population, a vessel, the **ramus intermedius**, arises from the **LCA** between the **LAD** and the **LCx**.

LAD: This travels down the **left interventricular groove**, reaching the apex in 78 per cent of the population. As well as supplying the anterolateral myocardium, interventricular septum and apex, it also typically supplies 45–55 per cent of the LV. Septal branches run perpendicular to the heart surface, perforating and supplying the interventricular septum. Diagonal branches run over the surface of the heart, supplying the lateral wall of the LV and the anterolateral papillary muscle.

LCx: This travels across the AV groove and gives off obtuse marginal branches. It supplies the **SA nodal artery** in 40 per cent of people (the RCA does this in the remaining 60 per cent of the population). It supplies 15–25 per cent of the LV in right-dominant systems, and 50 per cent in left-dominant systems.

RCA: Originating above the right cusp of the aortic valve, the RCA traverses the AV groove. It primarily supplies the RV and approximately 25–35 per cent of the LV. In 85 per cent of patients, the RCA gives rise to the posterior descending artery, which goes on to supply the inferior wall, ventricular septum and posteromedial papillary muscle. In 12–13 per cent of the population, the posterior descending artery arises from the circumflex artery.

39. In clinical practice, ECG changes are used to suggest the most likely site of cardiac pathology. This is particularly helpful in MI, as it can provide crucial information on the coronary vessels and heart walls involved. Using all of the labels provided, annotate the blank ECG to show both the coronary vessel(s) and heart wall(s) represented by each ECG lead

Almost always there should be a negative QRS complex in aVR. If this is not the case, suspect incorrect lead placement or dextrocardia. Other than this, aVR is generally of little diagnostic significance

I	aVR	V1	V4
II	aVL	V2	V5
III	aVF	V3	V6

Heart wall:
  Anterolateral
  Inferior
  Septal
  Lateral

Coronary vessel:
  Left anterior descending artery
  Left circumflex artery
  Right coronary artery

LCA, left coronary artery; RCA, right coronary artery; LAD, left anterior descending; LCx, left circumflex; AV, atrioventricular; SA, sinoatrial

EXPLANATION: ANATOMY AND TERRITORIES OF THE CORONARY ARTERIES (II)

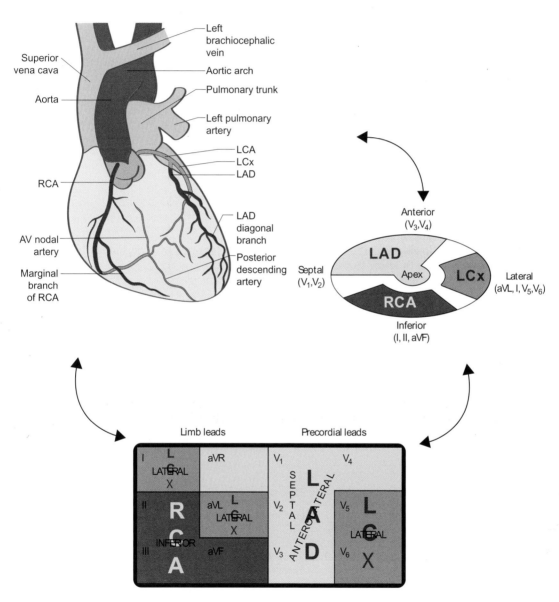

The relationship between ECG leads, heart walls and coronary arteries

---

Answer

39. See diagram

Consider the following features of arrhythmias and answer questions 40–43.
- **A.** Cardiac or non-cardiac
- **B.** Automaticity or re-entry
- **C.** Supraventricular or ventricular
- **D.** Bradycardia or tachycardia
- **E.** Irregular, regularly irregular or irregularly irregular
- **F.** Narrow complex (<0.12 seconds) or broad complex (>0.12 seconds) tachycardia

40. Match the above features to the most suitable category

Options

1. Mechanism
2. Origin
3. QRS complex
4. Rate
5. Cause
6. Rhythm

41. Match the following possible diagnoses to the two features of arrhythmias that you would most like to know to make that diagnosis

Options

1. Atrial fibrillation
2. Bradycardia due to hypothyroidism
3. Ventricular tachycardia
4. Wolff–Parkinson–White syndrome
5. Atrial flutter

42. Which of the following tools would be most useful in deciphering the difference between features in each of the categories of arrhythmia? You can suggest more than one

Options

1. Examination
2. History
3. ECG
4. Adenosine

43. Name three non-pharmacological ways of slowing the AV node

AV, atrioventricular; SVT, supraventricular tachycardia; AF, atrial fibrillation; VT, ventricular tachycardia

EXPLANATION: ARRHYTHMIAS

Recognizing arrhythmias starts as early as the history and examination. When patients describe feeling palpitations, ask them to tap them out or describe what they feel. An irregular tapping is more suggestive of fibrillation than the fast, regular 'fluttering' of other arrhythmias. Bradycardia or extrasystoles may give the sensation of missing out beats or even a 'thump', 'jump' or 'jolt' as the next beat is felt.

Arrhythmias may be categorized according to the following features (40)

Cause	Cardiac or non-cardiac
Mechanism	Automaticity or re-entry
Origin	Supraventricular or ventricular
Rate	Bradycardia or tachycardia
Rhythm	Regular, regularly irregular or irregularly irregular
QRS complex	Acute arrhythmias can be narrow complex (<0.12 seconds) or broad complex (>0.12 seconds) tachycardias

Other clues in the history include shortness of breath and syncope. The **cause** may also be identified; ask about previous cardiovascular disease, recent chest infections and thyroid disease. Quantify smoking, alcohol and caffeine intake. On **examination**, the pulse reveals the rate and rhythm.

Tachycardias (>100 bpm)	Bradycardias (<60 bpm)
SVTs	Second-degree AV block, Mobitz type I or Wenckebach, Mobitz type II, **regularly irregular**
AF, **irregularly irregular**	Third-degree block or complete AV block, **irregularly irregular**
Atrial flutter, **regular**	Absolute bradycardia (<40 bpm may be due to sick sinus syndrome; exclude drugs and hypothyroidism, **regular or irregular**
AV node re-entrant tachycardia, **regularly irregular**	
AV re-entrant tachycardia, **regularly irregular** *VTs*	
Ventricular fibrillation, **regular** Ventricular flutter	

Investigations such as **ECG** can show the type of arrhythmia. Ascertain the rate and rhythm, then identify P waves and their relationship to the QRS. Look at the width of the QRS interval, especially in patients with tachycardia. Specific clues from the ECG include a short PR interval in Wolff–Parkinson–White syndrome, a long QT interval due to hyperkalaemia, drugs or other metabolic disturbance, and U waves indicating hypokalaemia. Further investigations include electrolyte levels, exercise ECG or 24-hour tape, echocardiography and cardiac catheterization.

Appropriate treatment may be determined by the origin and **mechanism** of the arrhythmia. Conversely, some treatments are used to reveal underlying rhythms and thereby confirm the diagnosis. A response to **adenosine** can distinguish between narrow complex tachycardias. **Carotid sinus massage** slows sinus tachycardia and the ventricular response in AF and abruptly terminates paroxysmal SVT, but has no effect on VT. Other vagal manoeuvres to transiently increase AV block include the Valsalva manoeuvre and plunging the face into cold water. In extreme or symptomatic bradycardia, intravenous atropine, isoprenaline or temporary pacing via external pacing or insertion of a temporary pacing wire may be indicated.

Answers

40. See table

41. 1 – D (tachycardia) E (irregularly irregular), 2 – A (non-cardiac) D (bradycardia), 3 – C (ventricular) D (tachycardia), 4 – B (re-entry) F (narrow complex widened due to δ wave – see page 65), 5 – B (automaticity) E (regular)

42. 1 – ADE, 2 – A, 3 – BCDEF, 4 – BC

43. Carotid sinus massage, face in cold water, Valsalva manoeuvre

A 73-year-old woman who has returned from visiting her new grandson in Australia is seen in
A&E with a 2-hour history of palpitations and dyspnoea. She has a cough and has smoked 15
cigarettes per day for 50 years. She has a heart rate of 170 bpm, an irregularly irregular pulse
and a BP of 110/70 mmHg.

44. What are the most important steps in her initial management?

45. With reference to her electrocardiogram, answer the following questions

a. What does the electrocardiogram show?
b. What is happening in the atria?
c. What are the four main causes of this
   abnormal cardiac rhythm?
d. What other possible causes might you
   consider in this woman?

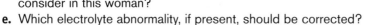

e. Which electrolyte abnormality, if present, should be corrected?
f. What is the most dangerous side-effect of this rhythm and how does it arise?

**46. There are three aspects of treatment of AF: (i) control of ventricular rate, (ii)
restoration of sinus rhythm and (iii) prevention of embolism**

a. For each one, suggest an appropriate drug
b. What is the target International Normalized Ratio and how is it achieved?
c. For each drug, mention an important or unwanted side-effect
d. What is the evidence concerning rate control versus rhythm control?
e. What treatments would you consider in this patient?

Another 73-year-old woman arrives in A&E. She has sliced her hand with a Stanley knife while
cutting out a cardboard base for a cake. At first glance, you can see that a few sutures or Steri-
Strips will deal with the cut. You take her pulse, which is about 80 bpm and irregularly irregular.
You tell her that her pulse is irregular and she seems surprised; she was unaware of this, takes
no medication and is not haemodynamically compromised.

47. With reference to the second case, answer the following short-answer questions

a. How do you know whether the atrial fibrillation is persistent or paroxysmal?
b. What investigations would you like to do?
c. If the decision is made to accept permanent atrial fibrillation, which treatments should
   be started?

AF, atrial fibrillation; AV, atrioventricular; PE, pulmonary embolism; COPD, chronic obstructive pulmonary disease; S1, first heart sound; INR,
International Normalized Ratio

EXPLANATION: ATRIAL FIBRILLATION

AF is the most common cardiac arrhythmia and is characterized by an **irregularly irregular** heartbeat. Atrial contraction is poorly coordinated and thus there are no P waves. It can be acute, chronic or paroxysmal.

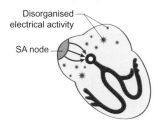
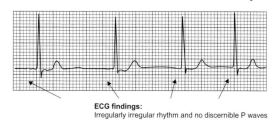

ECG findings:
Irregularly irregular rhythm and no discernible P waves

The underlying pathophysiology involves irregular impulses running in multiple wavelets in the atria occurring at a rate of 300–600 bpm. The AV node is continually bombarded, but due to its longer conduction and refractory times it randomly conducts at less than 200 bpm. The intermittent response of the AV node produces the irregularly irregular ventricular beat. Interestingly, the ventricular response is slower in diseases of the conducting system, in the elderly, and with beta-blockers, digoxin or a calcium channel blocker. The QRS complex may appear broad on the ECG if there is associated left or right bundle branch block.

The causes are largely cardiac, metabolic or pulmonary, and include **ischaemic heart disease**, **hypertension**, **mitral valve disease**, pericarditis, cardiomyopathy, left ventricular hypertrophy, **thyrotoxicosis**, alcohol, PE, COPD, cor pulmonale and pneumonia.

Signs and symptoms include dyspnoea, palpitations and chest pain. Patients may notice that their pulse is irregular. On examination, pulse character and volume can change from beat to beat, and S1 is of variable intensity. Signs of thyrotoxicosis, DVT or mitral stenosis may give clues to the underlying cause. BP and ECG should be recorded. Relevant blood tests include U&Es, troponin and thyroid function tests. Echocardiography may reveal structural damage or mitral valve disease.

Restoration of sinus **rhythm** can be achieved by amiodarone flecainide **(46a(ii))** or **DC cardioversion**. The emphasis on the use of drugs to control rhythm has been lost in recent years, as **rate** control is equally if not more important to survival **(46d)**. The main side-effect of anti-arrhythmic drugs is arrhythmias **(46c)**. **Digoxin** 500 micrograms/12 h is given for the first day, then 62.5–250 micrograms daily. A low-dose **beta-blocker** such as metoprolol 50 mg b.d. can be started to bring the heart rate down to 70–80 bpm **(46a(i))**.

INR refers to the prothrombin time and is a measurement of the time it takes for clotting via the extrinsic pathway in an individual compared with the rest of the population.

In patients with acute AF, **warfarin (46a(iii))** is used before and after DC cardioversion to reduce the associated risk of embolus. In patients with chronic AF, the risk of thrombus formation due to long-term stasis in the left atrium **(45f)** can be targeted by using **warfarin** titrated to an **INR** of 2.5–3.5 **(46b)**.

Answers

44. Airway, breathing, circulation, oxygen (high flow initially, but monitor arterial blood gases)

45. a – AF, b – See diagram, c – Ischaemic heart disease, hypertension, mitral valve disease and thyrotoxicosis, d – PE, pneumonia, COPD, alcohol, e – K$^+$, f – See explanation

46. a–d – See explanation, e – Control ventricular rate, anticoagulate with warfarin/aspirin, outpatient DC cardioversion

47. a – 24-hour tape, b – ECG, CXR, echocardiography, thyroid function tests, c – Digoxin $\pm$ beta-blocker plus warfarin titrated to target INR 2.5–3.5

48. Of the following arrhythmias, which would you class as narrow complex tachycardias?

    a. Atrial fibrillation
    b. Torsade de pointes
    c. Atrial flutter
    d. Atrioventricular nodal re-entry tachycardia
    e. Ventricular ectopics

49. In the following tachycardias, you would expect to see a normal P wave (true or false)

    a. Sinus tachycardia
    b. Supraventricular tachycardia
    c. Atrial fibrillation
    d. Junctional tachycardia
    e. Wolff–Parkinson–White syndrome

AF, atrial fibrillation; AV, atrioventricular; AVRT, atrioventricular re-entry tachycardia; AVNRT, atrioventricular node re-entry tachycardia

EXPLANATION: NARROW COMPLEX TACHYCARDIA (I)

This is defined as a tachycardia (rate >100 bpm) with ECG QRS complexes narrower than 3 small squares, indicating that each QRS lasts less than 0.12 seconds.

Sinus tachycardia: This is characterized by a fast rate but regular rhythm with normal underlying mechanisms. It occurs as a normal response to exercise and may be present in patients due to a drug or metabolic disturbance. ECG appears normal and P waves are present. Adenosine and vagal manoeuvres may slow the rate; however, the best management is to identify and treat the underlying cause.

Supraventricular tachycardias: These are more dangerous, as they may lead to ventricular tachycardia. ECG shows absent P waves or P waves inverted lying after the QRS complex. Acute management includes vagal manoeuvres and IV adenosine, which slow the rhythm. Irregular narrow complex tachycardias do not respond directly to adenosine; rather, the underlying flutter or fibrillation may be unmasked.

Atrial flutter: This has a characteristic 'saw-tooth' baseline, but unlike AF the beats that reach the ventricles have a regular rhythm and the rate is usually a factor of 300 bpm; for example, 2:1 AV block produces a rate of 150 bpm. Carotid sinus massage or IV adenosine transiently blocks the AV node, and may unmask the flutter and produce a greater ratio of block. Atrial flutter can be treated in a similar manner to AF. However, cavotricuspid isthmus ablation is a very effective definitive curative procedure and is increasingly offered.

Junctional tachycardias: These involve the AV node or bundle of His. AVRT and AVNRT result from impulses moving through the node at different rates. AVNRT and AVRT are therefore likely to be influenced by vagal manoeuvres and abolished by adenosine. Medical therapies include beta-blockers and amiodarone. Radiofrequency ablation is also used, particularly for AVRT if the arrhythmias recur.

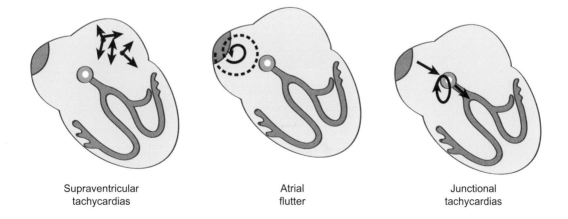

Supraventricular
tachycardias

Atrial
flutter

Junctional
tachycardias

Answers

48. a, c, d
49. T F F (absent) F (buried in QRS or after QRS) T (but PR interval shortened)

50. How would you give adenosine and what side effects would you warn the patient about?

51. For the following ECG examples, give (a) the rate, (b) the type of arrhythmia, (c) the response to adenosine that you would expect and (d) the treatment that you would recommend

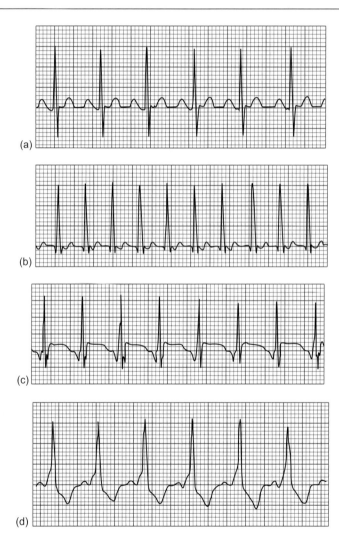

(a)

(b)

(c)

(d)

EXPLANATION: NARROW COMPLEX TACHYCARDIA (II)

Adenosine is a useful drug for patients with acute tachycardia as it works quickly and for a short time **(51)**; it also aids in making a diagnosis and is a form of treatment. Disadvantages include the fact that it will not treat atrial fibrillation or flutter, and has several side effects and contraindications. Warn patients that they may feel transient chest pain, which may be accompanied by headache or shortness of breath, and that they may become flushed **(50)**. Adenosine is usually given as an intravenous bolus in 6 or 12 mg volumes **(50)**.

A conduction pathway between the atria and the ventricles that is extra or accessory to the atrioventricular node can lead to arrhythmias. These can be congenital or acquired. The congenital form is known as Wolff–Parkinson–White syndrome and has a characteristic ECG with a shortened PR interval and δ waves. Patients may present with a regular or irregular narrow complex tachycardia. The best treatment would be to ablate the accessory pathway **(51)**.

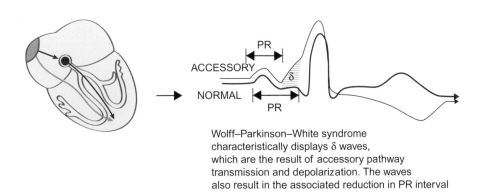

Wolff–Parkinson–White syndrome characteristically displays δ waves, which are the result of accessory pathway transmission and depolarization. The waves also result in the associated reduction in PR interval

Answers

50. See explanation
51. a – 125 bpm, 200 bpm, 150 bpm, 125 bpm, b – (i) Sinus tachycardia (ii) Supraventricular tachycardia (iii) Atrioventricular node re-entry tachycardia (iv) Wolf–Parkinson–White syndrome c–d – See explanation

52. The following are features of broad complex tachycardias (true or false)

a. QRS complexes are >0.12 seconds long
b. Are always ventricular in origin
c. May involve fusion beats and capture beats
d. Usually respond to intravenous adenosine
e. Electrocardiography shows right axis deviation

53. Give a short description of the following ECG findings

a. Monomorphic
b. Polymorphic
c. Concordance
d. Fusion beats
e. Capture beats

VT, ventricular tachycardia; VF, ventricular fibrillation; AF, atrial fibrillation; SVT, supraventricular tachycardia; S1, first heart sound

EXPLANATION: BROAD COMPLEX TACHYCARDIA (I)

Broad complex tachycardia is defined as a tachycardia (rate >100 bpm) with ECG QRS complexes broader than 3 small squares, indicating that each QRS lasts less than 0.12 seconds. These arrhythmias are generally more dangerous than narrow complex tachycardias. The differential diagnosis includes arrhythmias of ventricular origin (VT, ventricular ectopics, VF and torsades de pointes). However, it also includes arrhythmias that have a supraventricular origin associated with AF or atrial flutter, such as Wolff–Parkinson–White syndrome. Bundle branch block is a type of **aberrant** conduction through the atrioventricular node and causes an SVT to appear broad.

When attempting to differentiate between SVT and VT, go back to the history and examination. VT is more likely to be associated with a history of ischaemic heart disease or congestive cardiac failure. On examination, there may be 'cannon' waves in the jugular veins and variable intensity of S1. On the ECG, look at the length of the QRS. VT is much more likely in right bundle branch block with a QRS of more than 0.14 seconds or left bundle branch block with a QRS of more than 0.16 seconds (or 4 small squares). You should always assume that a broad complex tachycardia is VT, unless there is very convincing evidence to the contrary. Since such evidence is rarely available (e.g. a previous ECG showing sinus rhythm and identical bundle branch block), you should expect in almost all cases to treat the patient for VT.

Monomorphic VT shows repeating ventricular ectopics with very similar beat-to-beat morphology, and is the most common appearance of VT **(53a)**. Conversely, in **polymorphic** tachycardia the beats are very different in the appearance of the QRS complex and more likely to be supraventricular in origin **(53b)**. **Concordance** simply means that the QRS complexes point in the same direction **(53c)**. The figure shows how a ventricular focus may lead to a broad complex tachycardia; this is a common mechanism of VF.

Fusion and capture beats are both features of VT and occur when independent atrial beats are conducted to the ventricles. **Fusion** beats occur when a wave of depolarization travelling down from the atria occurs simultaneously with a wave of depolarization travelling up from the ventricular focus **(53d)**. **Capture** beats are normal QRS complexes occurring during VT **(53e)**.

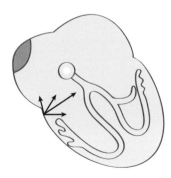

Answers
52. T F T F F
53. See explanation

54. For the following ECG examples, name (a) the rate and (b) the type of arrhythmia, and (c) give a brief description of what is happening

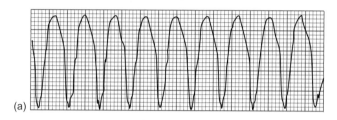

(a)

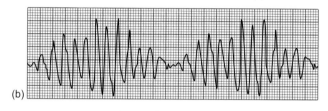

(b)

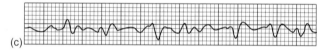

(c)

55. You are working in A&E when a patient is brought in by ambulance. He is a 76-year-old man who has collapsed in the street. His carotid pulse is absent and the paramedics are performing cardiac massage

    a. What are the five most important steps in the initial management?
    b. What potentially reversible causes would you like to exclude?
    c. His ECG is shown below. What is this rhythm?
    d. What difference does this make to what you can do to treat him?
    e. What treatment would you administer to cardiovert this rhythm?

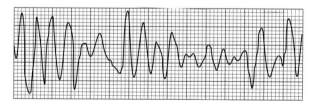

VT, ventricular tachycardia; VF, ventricular fibrillation; AF, atrial fibrillation

EXPLANATION: BROAD COMPLEX TACHYCARDIA (II)

Torsade de pointes is a type of polymorphic VT characterized by a continuously changing QRS vector **(54 (ii))**. It can occur in patients with the rare congenital long QT syndromes, but is more likely to be due to anti-arrhythmic drugs, electrolyte imbalance (especially K^+ and Mg^{2+}) or cardioactive drugs such as antidepressants, anti-arrhythmic drugs or phenothiazines. Treatment is to stop any causative agents and correct electrolyte imbalances.

If the origin of the tachycardia is unclear (ventricular versus supraventricular), it should be treated as VT. VT is relatively regular in rhythm, but can degenerate into VF, which is irregular, inefficient and likely to lead to cardiac arrest **(54 (iii))**. If in doubt, the patient should be treated as an emergency on the basis of the signs and symptoms; by following protocols, the safest treatment can be given (see Appendix, page 127).

It is important to assess the patient rather than relying on ECG findings. Adverse signs include chest pain, heart failure, systolic blood pressure below 90 mmHg and heart rate above 150 bpm. If the patient is well, anti-arrhythmic therapy is indicated. If a pulse is felt but the patient has adverse signs, or anti-arrhythmic therapy has failed, expert help and cardioversion are required. If the patient has no pulse, attempt defibrillation. VF, polymorphic VT, torsade de pointes and AF with pre-excitation all produce an irregular broad complex fast rhythm. These rhythms all have a high mortality, and fortunately defibrillation is the optimal treatment for all of them in the emergency situation. It is still useful to record the ECG to help in deciding on subsequent treatment.

Answers

54. a, b – (i) VT (ii) torsade de pointes (iii) VF, c – See explanation
55. a – Airway (call anaesthetist, intubate), breathing (high-flow oxygen), circulation (IV access, take bloods, give fluids, attach ECG, CPR; see Appendix, page 127), b – Hypoxia, hypovolaemia, hypothermia, hyperkalaemia, tension pneumothorax, cardiac tamponade, toxic agents, thromboembolic obstruction, c – VF, d – It is a shockable rhythm, e – Defibrillate using 360 kJ

ECG POINTERS

Ten simple points to cover when looking at an ECG:

- Check the patient details on the ECG (name, age and sex)
- What is the rate?
- Is the tracing in sinus rhythm?
- Is there deviation of the axis?
- Are the P waves normal? (look at lead II)
- Is the PR interval normal? (<5 small squares)
- Are the QRS complexes normal? (widened/left or right bundle branch block/left ventricular hypertrophy)
- Are the ST segments normal? (depressed/elevated)
- Are the T waves normal? (tented/flattened/inverted)
- Are there any abnormal U waves?

EXPLANATION: LEFT BUNDLE BRANCH BLOCK Cont'd from page 53

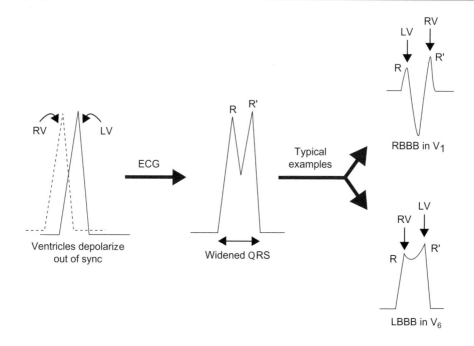

5 CONDITIONS

---

1. A 68-year-old man comes to A&E complaining of crushing central chest pain

    a. What questions would you specifically need to ask in the history?
    b. What might you expect to find on examination?
    c. Which initial investigation would you request and what questions would you want it to answer?

The man tells you that he has had severe central crushing chest pain lasting for 45 minutes. It also goes down his left arm. He has tried taking his GTN spray, which normally works for his angina, but this time it is not helping. He is feeling nauseous. He has had angina for the last 3 years, he takes regular medication for his BP, he has smoked 20 cigarettes per day for the last 30 years, and his father died aged 60 years from a heart attack. He does not have diabetes. On examination, he looks pale and sweaty. His pulse is 150 bpm, BP 170/90 mmHg, temperature 37.5 °C and respiratory rate 18/minute.

    d. What blood tests would you ask for and when?

This is his ECG.

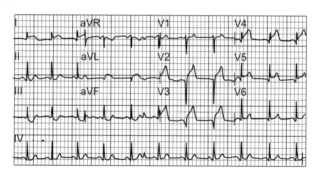

    e. What is your diagnosis now?
    f. What is your management plan now?
    g. In your hospital, the protocol is for a pharmacological approach. What further questions would you ask and what information would you need to give your patient before you take the next steps?
    h. The patient informs you that he underwent hemicolectomy last week for resection of colorectal carcinoma. How would this influence your management?
    i. A day later, you go to review your patient, who is now on the coronary care unit. What medications would you expect to find on the drug chart?

---

2. He asks you how long he is going to be in hospital. What do you tell him?

ACS, acute coronary syndrome; NSTEMI, non-ST elevation myocardial infarction; STEMI, ST elevation myocardial infarction

EXPLANATION: ACUTE CORONARY SYNDROMES (I)

'**Acute coronary syndrome**' is an umbrella term for three clinical entities: **unstable angina**, **NSTEMI** and **STEMI**. The diagnosis is made on the basis of the ECG and serum levels of cardio-specific proteins, troponins, which represent the extent of myocardial damage. Mortality from ACS is related to the territory of the infarction and correlates with ECG changes. ST elevation is associated with the highest risk, followed by ST depression and then T wave inversion. Mortality from acute STEMI is 4.5–25 per cent.

Pathophysiology

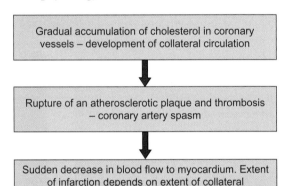

Gradual accumulation of cholesterol in coronary vessels – development of collateral circulation

Rupture of an atherosclerotic plaque and thrombosis – coronary artery spasm

Sudden decrease in blood flow to myocardium. Extent of infarction depends on extent of collateral circulation and superimposed vasospasm

Complications

- Further episodes: 8 per cent of patients with ACS suffer re-infarction
- Cardiac arrest/cardiogenic shock
- Heart failure
- Pericarditis
- Arrythmias (tachy/brady/heart block)
- Systemic embolism: stroke, DVT/pulmonary embolism
- Other cardiac damage: mitral regurgitation, ventricular septal defect, LV aneurysm, cardiac tamponade
- Dressler's syndrome: recurrent pericarditis, pleural effusions, fever, anaemia and raised ESR one to three weeks post-MI (treat with NSAIDs/ corticosteroids).

In retrospect, STEMI is diagnosed when there are **both ST segment changes on the ECG and elevated cardiac markers in serum**. When a patient presents, however, immediate diagnosis of STEMI can be made on the symptoms and ST elevation. It is important *not* to delay for blood tests. When ST elevation is present on the ECG the patient should be transferred for **immediate emergency coronary angiography and intervention (1f)** or, where this is unavailable, should receive **thrombolysis**. Before giving thrombolysis ask the patient about contraindications (principally active bleeding, surgery within last two weeks **(1h)**, haemorrhagic stroke, pregnancy) and warn about the risk of stroke **(1g)**.

Characteristics of the three acute coronary syndromes are tabulated in the Appendix, page 126.

Answers

1. a–b – See explanation on page 75, c – See explanation on page 77, d – STEMI, e–h – See explanation, also on page 77, i – See explanation on page 77
2. Average length of stay is about 1 week

3. Which ONE of the statements below BEST describes the condition of unstable angina?

a. Chest pain at rest

b. Chest pain on minimal exertion or at rest, increasing in frequency and severity over a few weeks, associated with non-specific electrocardiogram changes

c. Chest pain on minimal exertion or at rest, increasing in frequency and severity over a few weeks with no associated changes on the electrocardiogram but evidence of myocardial damage in the form of elevated cardiac enzymes

d. Chest pain on minimal exertion or at rest, increasing in frequency and severity over a few weeks with no dynamic changes on the electrocardiogram or elevations in cardiac markers of myocardial necrosis

4. Answer the following statements as true or false

a. Unstable angina is not associated with an increased risk of further cardiovascular events

b. Non-ST elevation myocardial infarction can be diagnosed only once the 12-hour troponin result has returned showing elevated levels

c. Elderly patients and those with diabetes always present with typical symptoms of myocardial infarction

d. Aortic dissection can present in a similar manner to ST segment myocardial infarction and requires similar management

e. Thrombolysis is indicated when electrocardiography shows ST elevation, posterior myocardial infarction or right bundle branch block

5. Which treatments are proven to reduce mortality from ACS? True or false

a. Angiotensin-converting enzyme inhibitors

b. Beta-blockers

c. Aspirin

d. Aspirin plus clopidogrel

e. Statins

f. Coronary revascularization

6. Regarding the pathophysiology of ACS

a. Acute coronary syndrome is due to gradual occlusion of a coronary artery

b. The extent of an infarct may be determined by the presence of a collateral circulation

c. Vasospasm does not play a role in acute coronary syndrome

d. Atheromatous plaque rupture with thrombosis is the commonest cause of acute infarction

---

ACS, acute coronary syndrome; PE, pulmonary embolism; S4, fourth heart sound; S3, third heart sound

EXPLANATION: ACUTE CORONARY SYNDROMES (II)

In the **history**, it is essential to ask about **(1a)**:

- Duration of pain and relief by nitrates
- Risk factors for ischaemic heart disease (smoking, hypertension, diabetes, hyperlipidaemia, family history)
- Past history of angina/MI/peripheral vascular disease/cerebrovascular disease
- Symptoms of aortic dissection (tearing pain through to back, collapse).

Characteristically, acute MI presents with central, crushing chest pain radiating to the left arm/jaw. It has an acute onset of several minutes and lasts **at least 30 minutes**. It is *not* relieved by sublingual GTN. Fifty per cent of patients are woken from sleep with chest pain. Associated symptoms include sweating, nausea, vomiting, a sense of impending doom, breathlessness and palpitations. Unstable angina is characterized by a short history (weeks) of angina attacks of increasing frequency, severity and duration occurring on **minimal exertion or at rest**, only partially relieved by GTN. **Elderly patients and those with diabetes** may present atypically; for example, with unusual localization of pain or syncope.

Remember to ask questions to exclude differential diagnoses such as **aortic dissection**, **pericarditis**, **PE**, **pneumonia** and **ruptured peptic ulcer**.

Examination is often normal **(1b)**, but it is important to determine whether the patient is **haemodynamically stable** and whether there are signs of any other differentials; for example, progressive loss of peripheral pulses in aortic dissection, signs of a chest infection or marked tachycardia in PE.

Signs suggestive of ACS include:

- Pallor, sweating, apprehension
- Sinus tachycardia (bradycardia may develop if there is heart block), hypotension may indicate cardiogenic shock
- Precordium: area of dyskinesia, audible S4 (transient), audible S3 (indicates severe LV dysfunction)
- Respiratory signs: signs of respiratory distress, end-inspiratory crackles may be present, frank pulmonary oedema may be present in extensive anterior infarction.

Look for evidence of cardiovascular risk factors such as hypertension and hypertensive retinopathy, tendon xanthomata, ocular xanthelasma, corneal arcus and tar staining of fingers. Also look for signs of peripheral vascular disease: cool peripheries and absent pulses.

Answers

3. d
4. F T F F F (LBBB)
5. T (most benefit in elderly or LV dysfunction) T T T T T
6. F (sudden occlusion) T F T

7. Summary of approach to ACS: 'fill in the gaps'

Immediate management of all patients with severe chest pain:

    a

    b

    c

    d

    e

    f

Initial investigations:

    g

    h

    i

    j

Further management:

    If electrocardiogram shows ST elevation: **k**

    If electrocardiogram shows no ST elevation: **l**

Diagnosis:

    If 12-hour troponin is raised: **m**

    If 12-hour troponin is not raised: **n**

8. Regarding thrombolysis, answer true or false

    a. Pregnancy is an absolute contraindication to thrombolytic therapy

    b. Once patients have been given streptokinase, they must always receive streptokinase again in any future thrombolytic therapy

    c. Tissue plasminogen activator is less effective than streptokinase

    d. There is a 5 per cent risk of stroke with thrombolysis

    e. Thrombolysis is most effective if given 12 hours after the occlusive vascular event

---

ACS, acute coronary syndrome; CK, creatine kinase; CK-MB, creatinine kinase, myocardial enzyme; LDH, lactate dehydrogenase; PTCA, percutaneous transluminal coronary angioplasty; STEMI, ST elevation myocardial infarction; tPA, tissue plasminogen activator; SK, streptokinase

EXPLANATION: ACUTE CORONARY SYNDROMES (III)

Initial investigations **(7g, i, j)** for suspected ACS include an **ECG (1c)** (ST elevation [highest risk of mortality], ST depression, T wave inversion) and **cardiac biomarkers** such as troponins **(1d)** (send blood sample for testing 12 hours after onset of chest pain) and other enzymes (CK, CK-MB, LDH). Other investigations include a **CXR** (may show cardiomegaly or evidence of cardiac failure such as pulmonary oedema **(7h)**); **echocardiography** (detects abnormal wall motion, reduced ejection fraction, valve abnormalities); and **coronary angiography** (may be required if the diagnosis is in doubt or as part of definitive treatment).

For immediate management: remember the acronym 'MONA' **(7a–f)**:

- Resuscitation: ABC, IV access
- **M**orphine: 10 mg IV
- **O**$_2$: 15 L/minute, mask and reservoir bag
- **N**itrates: sublingual/tablet
- **A**spirin: 300 mg chewed
- Beta-blockers: 5 mg IV atenolol may be given.

Further management **(1i, 7l)** is aimed at **relieving symptoms** (e.g. IV nitrates for persisting pain) and **reducing mortality**. Treatments proven to reduce mortality include **antiplatelet therapy**: aspirin and clopidogrel 75 mg o.d. (unless thromboylysis is performed), glycoprotein IIb/IIIa antagonists if PTCA is performed, **beta-blockers** (unless contraindicated), **statins, ACE inhibitors** and **anticoagulation** (heparin or LMWH until coronary angiography). **Modifiable risk factors** can be addressed, though the effect on mortality is not proven. The **DIGAMI regimen** (glucose, potassium and insulin) should be considered in diabetic patients to maximize glucose entry into cardiac myocyles.

The specific treatment for STEMI **(1e, 7k)** is either **primary angioplasty** or **thrombolysis**. Immediate ('primary') coronary angioplasty gives better survival outcomes than thrombolysis, because it mechanically displaces thrombus. Most hospitals provide a 24-hour emergency service for primary angioplasty in STEMI patients. Thrombolytic agents tPA and the more immunogenic but cheaper SK were the mainstays of treatment of STEMI in the 1980s and 1990s. They remain valuable in situtations where emergency angioplasty is unavailable, but should be given as soon as possible, preferably within 3 hours. There are a number of disadvantages associated with thrombolysis including a 1 per cent risk of stroke and a reduced chance of successful revascularization. Patients who have already received SK in the past cannot be given it a second time.

Answers

7. a–l – See explanation, m – STEMI or NSTEMI, n – Unstable angina
8 F F F F F

9. A 62-year-old retired bus driver presents to his GP complaining of repeated episodes of chest pain when digging in his garden. He has known hypertension and smokes 20 cigarettes per day. He has a history of peptic ulcer disease.

    a. What is your differential diagnosis?

    b. What other questions would you ask in the history?

    c. What might you expect to find on examination?

    d What investigations would you ask for?

    e How would you manage this patient initially?

    f What features would make you more concerned about the nature of patient's underlying pathology?

10. Regarding the pathophysiology underlying angina pectoris: true or false?

    a. Myocardial ischaemia is caused by an imbalance in myocardial oxygen demand and supply

    b. Most angina symptoms are produced when coronary arteries are occluded by atherosclerotic plaque rupture

    c. Vasospasm has no role in causing angina in the presence of diseased coronary arteries

    d. Printzmetal's variant angina is not relieved by glyceryl trinitrate

    e. Aortic stenosis may predispose a patient to angina symptoms

11. What are the independent risk factors for coronary artery disease? True or false

    a. Excess alcohol consumption

    b. Hypotension

    c. Male gender

    d. Diabetes insipidus

    e. Cigarette smoking

    f. Body mass index greater than 24 kg/m^2

ACS, acute coronary syndrome; COPD, chronic obstructive pulmonary disease; PE, pulmonary embolism

EXPLANATION: ANGINA PECTORIS (I)

Angina pectoris is defined as **episodic chest pain** caused by **reversible myocardial ischaemia**. It can be differentiated from ACS by 1) its predictable onset in response to cardiac stress, 2) its duration (minutes rather than hours) and 3) its relief by nitrates. Most cases of angina are caused by arterial narrowing, whereas ACS is caused by sudden occlusion. However, new-onset angina may occur when one artery is blocked but at rest there is sufficient collateral flow, so pain occurs only on exertion. The annual mortality from disease of a single coronary artery is 1–2 per cent.

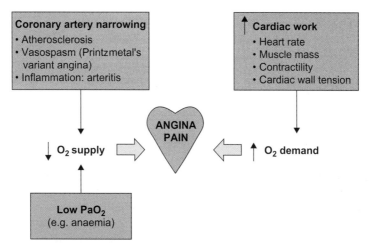

Angina can progress into an ACS **(13a)**; suspect if the patient begins to complain of **pain at rest, not relieved by GTN, lasting longer than 30 minutes**.

Essential information to gather in the **history (9b)**:

- Features distinguishing angina from ACS: (1) provoked by cardiac stressors such as **exertion**, **anxiety** or **smoking**, (2) **relieved by rest** or by administration of sublingual **nitrates**, (3) only lasts for a **few minutes**
- **Independent risk factors** for cardiovascular disease: male, age, family history, hypertension, diabetes mellitus, hyperlipidaemia, cigarette smoking
- Other possible differentials: for example, **cardiovascular**: history of anaemia or bleeding, arrhythmias, cardiac valve disease (e.g. aortic stenosis), **respiratory**: pneumothorax (?asthma/COPD), pneumonia, previous PE/DVT, **gastrointestinal**: gastritis, peptic ulcer disease
- Elicit how much the pain limits the patient's daily activities.

Examination is often normal **(9c)**, but you must look for **evidence of cardiovascular risk factors** (see page 73) and look for **signs of peripheral vascular disease** such as cold peripheries, absent pulses and arterial ulcers. There may be evidence of other medical conditions predisposing to angina: the pale conjunctiva of anaemia, the fast, irregularly irregular pulse of atrial fibrillation or the slow rising pulse of aortic stenosis.

Answers

9. a – ACS, angina pectoris, recurrent peptic ulcer disease, b–c – See explanation, d–e – See explanation on page 81, f – Features of ACS, syncope, ST/T wave changes on resting ECG
10. T F F F T (through LV hypertrophy and increased muscle mass)
11. F F T F T F

12. Regarding the treatment of angina pectoris: true or false?

a. Medical therapy does not improve long-term survival
b. Glyceryl trinitrate and isosorbide dinitrate relieve angina symptoms by reducing cardiac contractility
c. Aspirin is given to all patients with angina unless there are contraindications
d. Beta-blockers work in angina by increasing heart rate and reducing myocardial contractility
e. Coronary artery bypass grafting has similar mortality and morbidity to that of coronary angioplasty
f. Coronary artery bypass grafting tends to be reserved for patients in whom angioplasty is unlikely to achieve good revascularization
g. Stenting has helped to reduce the rate of restenosis after percutaneous transluminal coronary angioplasty

13. What are the major complications of

a. Angina pectoris
b. Coronary artery bypass grafting
c. Percutaneous transluminal coronary angioplasty

CABG, coronary artery bypass grafting; PTCA, percutaneous transluminal coronary angioplasty

EXPLANATION: ANGINA PECTORIS (II)

Specific investigations for suspected angina pectoris **(9d)** include:

- **Resting ECG**: often normal, but may show evidence of previous infarcts
- **Exercise treadmill test**: ECG changes occurring during the recovery period (maximal oxygen debt to the myocardium) and the time taken for the ECG to return to normal are sensitive indicators
- **Radionucleide scintigraphy**
- **Coronary angiography**: required for definitive diagnosis of coronary artery stenosis.

Medical management of angina pectoris follows a step-wise approach **(9e)**, adding in treatments as necessary.

Medical treatment proven to reduce mortality	Symptomatic treatment: reduce coronary artery tone	Address modifiable risk factors
Antiplatelet therapy: aspirin, clopidogrel **ACE inhibitors** **Lipid-lowering agents**: statins	**Nitrates**: GTN, isosorbide dinitrate/mononitrate (reduce vasospasm, directly cause coronary vasodilatation, redistribution of myocardial blood flow and collateral blood flow, and reduce preload and afterload on the heart) **Calcium channel antagonists**: diltiazem, amlodipine, nifedipine **Potassium channel openers**: Nicorandil	• Treat hypertension • Control blood glucose levels in diabetes • Stop smoking • Do more exercise • Eat a healthy diet • Reduce stress

Coronary revascularization is used in the definitive treatment of angina pectoris. There are two types of approach: **1) Coronary artery bypass grafting (CABG)** using internal mammary artery or saphenous vein grafts. After successful surgery, 75–90 per cent of patients are symptom free. Long-term prognosis is improved in patients with multiple-vessel disease. Perioperative mortality is 1–3 per cent. Perioperative complications include bleeding, wound infection, MI, stroke, atrial arrhythmia **(13b)**. Graft occlusion (higher risk with vein grafts than arterial grafts) is a late complication **(13b)**. **2) Coronary angioplasty/stenting (PTCA)**, where a guiding catheter is introduced via the femoral, brachial or radial artery. A balloon catheter is passed over a guide-wire in the stenosis and inflated to increase the luminal diameter. Restenosis occurs in 30 per cent of patients within six months. Placement of stents to hold the arteries open reduces the risk of restenosis to 15 per cent. Peri-intervention complications include bleeding, embolic stroke and arterial dissection **(13c)**. Late complications include restenosis and thrombosis of the stent **(13c)**. Most patients are better suited to PTCA, even those with triple-vessel disease. The long-term prognosis following PTCA is similar to that for CABG when similar patient groups are compared.

Answers

12. F F T F F (CABG has about 5–10 times higher peri-procedural mortality than angioplasty) T T
13. a – See explanation on page 79, b–c – See explanation

14. A 72-year-old woman presents with symptoms of chest pain and feeling dizzy on occasion. From the history, you elicit that she has always been a healthy individual. She does not have any risk factors for coronary heart disease apart from her age and she does not take any regular medication.

    a. What further areas do you specifically focus on in the history?
    b. What might you look for on examination?

On examination, the findings of note are a slow rising pulse and a systolic murmur.

    c. What characteristics are you expecting the murmur to have?
    d. What other findings might you expect on examination?
    e. What investigations would you request to confirm your suspected diagnosis?
    f. How would you manage this patient?
    g. If you had found the same murmur incidentally when the patient came to you for an unrelated sprained ankle, how would you manage her then?

15. Answer the following questions about aortic stenosis (true or false?)

    a. The classic triad of symptoms in aortic stenosis are 1) chest pain, 2) dyspnoea and 3) palpitations
    b. Aortic stenosis causes volume overload of the left ventricle
    c. Aortic stenosis produces a constellation of examination findings, including a wide pulse pressure, a collapsing pulse and a displaced apex beat
    d. Aortic stenosis produces a high-pitched ejection systolic murmur radiating to the carotids that may be associated with a systolic flow murmur and a low-pitched systolic murmur heard best at the mitral area
    e. In asymptomatic aortic stenosis with no evidence of left ventricular failure, the accepted management is to watch and wait

EXPLANATION: AORTIC STENOSIS (I)

Common causes

Nodular calcification of a
congential bicuspid valve,
usually presents in middle age

Diffuse calcification of a
trileaflet valve, usually presents
in old age. Occasionally it is due to
rheumatic heart disease, when it is
associated with mitral valve disease

 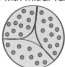

Pathophysiology

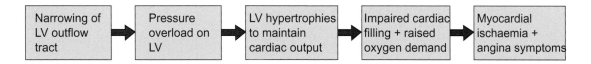

| Narrowing of LV outflow tract | ➡ | Pressure overload on LV | ➡ | LV hypertrophies to maintain cardiac output | ➡ | Impaired cardiac filling + raised oxygen demand | ➡ | Myocardial ischaemia + angina symptoms |

Complications of aortic stenosis include LV failure, myocardial ischaemia, infective endocarditis, thrombo-embolism (stroke, amaurosis fugax) and do not forget sudden death.

In the history, elicit the **classic triad** of symptoms and ask about **risk factors (14a)**:

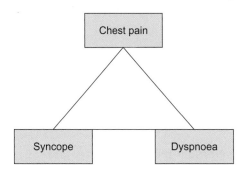

- Bicuspid valve
- Rheumatic fever
- High cholesterol
- Diabetes mellitus.

Answers

14. a–g – See explanation above and on page 85
15. F F F T T

16. Regarding the aetiology and pathophysiology of aortic stenosis, answer true or false

a. Aortic stenosis is most commonly caused by a bicuspid aortic valve
b. Rheumatic heart disease most commonly affects the aortic valve
c. Risk factors for senile calcification of the aortic valve include being female and having diabetes
d. Aortic stenosis causes early left ventricular dilatation
e. Impaired filling of the coronary arteries in aortic stenosis produces symptoms of angina

17. Which of the following are complications of aortic stenosis?

a. Arrhythmia
b. Sudden death
c. Aortic dissection
d. Myocardial ischaemia
e. Rheumatic fever

S2, second heart sound

EXPLANATION: AORTIC STENOSIS (II)

Peripheral signs of aortic stenosis **(14b)** include a **slow rising, low-volume pulse and narrow pulse pressure** (in severe cases). At the precordium, the **apex is not displaced** and there may be a **left parasternal heave** and a **systolic thrill (14d)**. On auscultation, there is an **ejection systolic murmur**, loudest in aortic area, that radiates to the carotids **(14c)**. In severe aortic stenosis, S2 becomes quiet.

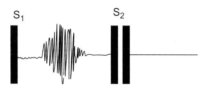

Ejection systolic murmur

Specific investigations (14e) include:

- **ECG**: LV strain
- **CXR**: normal cardiac size, post-stenotic dilatation of ascending aorta, valve calcification
- **Echocardiography**: required for **definitive diagnosis**; shows restricted valve leaflet motion and measures pressure gradient across valve (significance depends on cardiac output).

In **asymptomatic** patients **(14g)**, you can afford to '**watch and wait**', with six- to twelve-monthly echocardiography and antibiotic prophylaxis for prevention of infective endocarditis.

Surgery is indicated for **severe stenosis** (symptomatic **(14f)**, slow rising pulse, evidence of LV dysfunction on echocardiography, pressure gradient >50 mmHg across valve – though local guidelines vary). **Aortic valve replacement** is the main treatment. **Balloon aortic valvuloplasty** may be appropriate in young patients with a pliable valve.

After aortic valve replacement, **10-year survival has been reported as 70–75 per cent**. Balloon valvuloplasty produces an improvement in symptoms, but restenosis occurs within six to eighteen months in most cases. Development of symptoms immediately puts the patient in a poor prognostic category.

Answers

16. F F (mitral valve in 70 per cent of cases) F (male and diabetic) F T
17. a, b, d

18. **A 76-year-old man complains of shortness of breath when walking up stairs. On further questioning, the patient reveals that he also gets breathless in the middle of the night and has to go to the window for fresh air. He has generally been healthy in the past and is taking regular antihypertensive medication, though he admits that he sometimes forgets to take it**

    a. What is in your differential diagnosis?
    b. What further questions would you ask in the history?
    c. What salient features in the examination would you look for?

On examination, the patient's pulse appears to fall away from beneath your fingers at the radial and the brachial artery. His BP is 170/60 mmHg. On examination of the precordium, you feel the apex beat in the mid-axillary line and hear a mid-diastolic murmur on auscultation.

    d. What do you think the murmur represents?
    e. What are the characteristic features of this murmur and what other signs may accompany it?
    f. What investigations would you like to do?
    g. How would you manage this patient?
    h. What signs would indicate that his condition was becoming more severe?
    i. What might be the aetiology of this patient's condition?

19. **Regarding examination findings in AR**

    a. Aortic regurgitation may be associated with an ejection systolic murmur
    b. A low-pitched diastolic murmur heard at the apex represents the regurgitant jet of blood through the incompetent valve
    c. On examination of the periphery, you may expect to find a slow rising pulse
    d. From inspection at the end of the bed, a nodding head and visible carotid pulsations may give the diagnosis of aortic regurgitation
    e. The apex is never displaced

20. **Regarding management of AR, answer true or false**

    a. Surgery is not necessary until severe symptoms develop
    b. Antibiotic prophylaxis against infective endocarditis is not usually needed
    c. Tissue valves are preferred in young adults and children
    d. Diuretics should never be used in aortic regurgitation

AR, aortic regurgitation

EXPLANATION: AORTIC REGURGITATION

Common causes

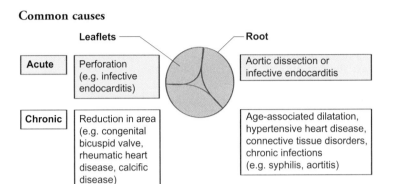

Leaflets — Root

Acute — Perforation (e.g. infective endocarditis) — Aortic dissection or infective endocarditis

Chronic — Reduction in area (e.g. congenital bicuspid valve, rheumatic heart disease, calcific disease) — Age-associated dilatation, hypertensive heart disease, connective tissue disorders, chronic infections (e.g. syphilis, aortitis)

Aortic regurgitation (AR) leads to **volume overload** of the LV. If acute, this can cause sudden low-output LV failure. Chronically, compensatory cardiac mechanisms maintain an adequate cardiac output until decompensation occurs.

When taking the history, determine whether there are **symptoms of LV failure** (exertional dyspnoea, orthopnoea, nocturnal dyspnoea) and exclude other causes of breathlessness. Find out **how the symptoms have progressed** over recent months and ask about **risk factors** (e.g. hypertension, aortic dissection, infections such as syphilis or rheumatic fever, connective tissue disorders, congenital valve abnormalities).

Peripheral signs of AR **(18c)** include a **collapsing pulse** and a **wide pressure**, as well as a long list of eponymous signs **(18e)** including Quincke's sign: visible nail bed pulsation; Corrigan's sign: carotid pulsation, pulsatile head nodding; de Musset's sign: pulsatile head nodding; Duroziez's sign: femoral diastolic murmur; Traube's sign: pistol shot sound over femoral arteries. Look for any **signs of cardiac failure (18h)** (displaced hyperdynamic apex, bibasal pulmonary crepitations). Auscultation reveals an **early diastolic murmur (18e)** (high pitched, loudest at left sternal edge and on sitting forwards at end-expiration). Other murmurs may also be heard, such as a **systolic flow murmur** across the aortic valve and the **Austin Flint murmur** (late rumbling diastolic murmur at apex due to regurgitant jet causing premature closure of mitral valve in diastole).

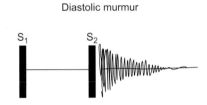

Diastolic murmur

S_1 S_2

Specific investigations (18f) include an **ECG** (LV strain pattern); **CXR** (cardiomegaly, dilated ascending aorta, pulmonary oedema if in LV failure); **Echocardiography** (an important prognostic indicator; shows an abnormally thickened aortic valve or dilated aortic root; Doppler can detect regurgitant jet). **Aortography** or **MRI** are recommended before surgical intervention.

Asymptomatic patients can be managed **conservatively**. However, once the ventricle has started to fail, it never fully recovers its function, even after surgery, therefore care must be taken not to watch and wait for too long. **Valve replacement (18g)** is indicated for severe regurgitation or evidence of LV dysfunction on echocardiography. **Mechanical valves** are used in most patients, as these last for decades. **Tissue valves** have the advantage of not requiring anticoagulation but often last for only a few years; they are therefore reserved for the very elderly and for women of reproductive age. If ventricular function is normal, aortic regurgitation is associated with a normal life span. Valve replacement at the right time can improve prognosis.

Answers

18. a – Cardiomyopathy, valve disease (e.g. AR), b – Seek risk factors for AR, exclude other causes of heart failure, c – See explanation, d – AR, e–h – See explanation, i – Chronic hypertension, age
19. T T F T F
20. F F F F

21. **A 48-year-old woman presents to her GP because of increasing fatigue and shortness of breath, and because today she experienced a sudden onset of sharp chest pain. The chest pain today came on suddenly and lasted only a few seconds. It was a sharp, stabbing pain and did not radiate. It left her feeling a little light-headed. She tells you that over the last few months she has been getting a 'funny sensation of a "whooshing"' of her heart. She has started using three pillows at night as she feels breathless when she lies flat. She has no other past medical history**

    a. What is in your differential diagnosis?
    b. What do you specifically look for in the examination?

On examination, you see a well looking woman. The only finding is a pansystolic murmur.

    c. What is your diagnosis?
    d. What are the characteristic signs associated with this murmur?
    e. What is the most likely aetiology of this patient's condition?
    f. What investigations would you like to do?
    g. How will you manage this patient?

22. **Regarding the aetiology and pathophysiology of MR, answer true or false**

    a. Chronic mitral regurgitation is often caused by papillary muscle rupture
    b. In acute mitral regurgitation, the left atrium distends so that pulmonary venous pressure does not rise significantly
    c. Mitral regurgitation may be caused by aortic valve disease
    d. Mitral regurgitation results in pressure overload of the left ventricle
    e. The left ventricle enlarges to accommodate the additional stroke volume collected in the left atrium through the regurgitant valve

23. **Regarding the management of MR, answer true or false**

    a. Serial echocardiography may be sufficient in asymptomatic patients
    b. Antibiotic prophylaxis against endocarditis is not needed
    c. Surgical valve repair or valve replacement is indicated if echocardiography shows progressive cardiac enlargement
    d. Acute mitral valve regurgitation cannot be treated surgically
    e. Surgical treatment is more effective the more the left ventricle is dilated

MR, mitral regurgitation; AF, atrial fibrillation; S3, third heart sound; S2, second heart sound

EXPLANATION: MITRAL REGURGITATION AND MITRAL VALVE PROLAPSE

Common causes and pathophysiology of MR

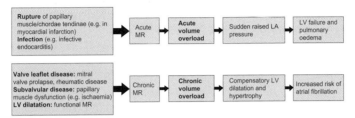

MR may be asymptomatic until the LV begins to fail, causing characteristic symptoms of **exertional fatigue and dyspnoea, orthopnoea or nocturnal dyspnoea**. Chronic MR can present with **palpitations** associated with AF. Ask about **risk factors** for MR such as previous MI, coronary artery disease or rheumatic fever.

On examination there may be an **irregularly irregular, low-volume pulse**. On palpation of the precordium, you may feel a **hyperdynamic displaced apex and systolic thrill** (only in severe MR). Auscultation characteristically reveals a **pansystolic murmur** radiating to the left axilla, sometimes associated with an S3, representing rapid filling of the dilated LV **(21d)**. Severe MR is indicated by the presence of **symptoms and signs of LV failure**, a **low-volume pulse**, a **long murmur** obscuring S2 and a **systolic click**.

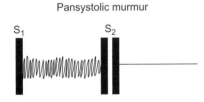

Pansystolic murmur

On an **ECG** AF is often present, but if not you might see a broad, bifid P wave (P mitrale) **(21f)**. The **CXR** may show cardiomegaly and/or a calcified mitral valve **(21f)**. **Echocardiography** confirms LA and LV dilatation and dynamic abnormalities of valve and valvular vegetations in endocarditis; Doppler detects the regurgitant jet in the LA and assesses the severity of the lesion **(21f)**.

Medical treatment of MR includes diuretics or ACE inhibitors for dyspnoea and antibiotic prophylaxis **(21g)** against infective endocarditis. **Surgery** is indicated for progressive symptoms of fatigue or dyspnoea or for echocardiographic evidence of LV dilatation **(21g)**. **Mitral valve reconstruction** is considered better than mitral valve replacement, though acute MR may require emergency valve replacement. MR is slowly progressive and associated with a **normal lifespan**. Once **LV failure develops**, life expectancy is **5–10 years**. The prognosis also depends on the aetiology, ischaemia being worse than rheumatic heart disease.

Mitral valve prolapse is caused by myxomatous degeneration of the valve leaflets and occurs in 5 per cent of the population, more commonly in women. It is associated with syndromes such as Turner's or Marfan's. It is often asymptomatic, but may present with atypical chest pain, palpitations or vague symptoms of anxiety, exercise intolerance or postural giddiness. On examination, you will hear a **mid-systolic click** followed by a **late systolic murmur**. Echocardiography is **diagnostic**, showing posterior displacement of the mitral valve immediately following the systolic click. Mitral valve prolapse is usually **managed conservatively** with explanation and reassurance, and advice to avoid stimulants. Small doses of **beta-blockers** may be used to treat palpitations **(21e, f)**.

Answers

21. a – Flow murmur, pulmonary embolism, musculoskeletal pain, mitral valve prolapse, b – Signs of heart failure, DVT, cardiac murmur, c – MR, d – See explanation, e – Mitral valve prolapse, f–g – See explanation

22. F F T F T

23. T F T F F (efficacy reduced in more advanced disease)

24. A 60-year-old Indian woman presents to A&E after collapsing in the street. She describes a six-month history of increasing breathlessness and cough productive of blood-stained sputum. Today, before the collapse, she remembers that her heart was beating very fast, and she taps out an irregular rhythm for you

    a. What is on your list of differential diagnoses?
    b. What signs would you look for on examination? What bedside tests might you do?

On examination, she is breathless and flushed in the cheeks. Her pulse is 120 bpm and irregularly irregular. Her JVP is raised at 3 cm. On palpation, you feel a tapping apex, and on auscultation you hear a diastolic murmur. There are crepitations in both lung bases.

    c. What do you think the murmur represents? What are its characteristic features?
    d. What key risk factor should you ask this woman about?
    e. What features on examination would indicate that the lesion is severe?
    f. What might you expect to see on the electrocardiogram?
    g. How would you manage this patient?

25. Regarding the aetiology and pathophysiology of mitral stenosis, answer true or false

    a. The commonest cause is rheumatic heart disease
    b. Rheumatic mitral stenosis is more common in men than in women
    c. Left atrial dilatation helps to reduce pulmonary hypertension initially
    d. Atrial contraction does not aid ventricular filling
    e. Atrial fibrillation is a complication of mitral stenosis and can cause a sudden reduction in cardiac output

26. Regarding the presentation of mitral stenosis, answer true or false

    a. Mitral stenosis presents with symptoms of chest pain and syncope
    b. Mitral stenosis might present as chronic bronchitis
    c. Cyanotic discoloration of the tongue may be seen in mitral stenosis
    d. An irregularly irregular pulse may be felt
    e. It may present with an enlarged, pulsatile liver

AF, atrial fibrillation; BM, Boehringer Mannheim (test); COPD, chronic obstructive pulmonary disease; S1, first heart sound; S2, second heart sound

EXPLANATION: MITRAL STENOSIS

By far the most common cause of mitral stenosis is **rheumatic fever**. It may take up to 20 years for mitral stenosis to develop following the infection.

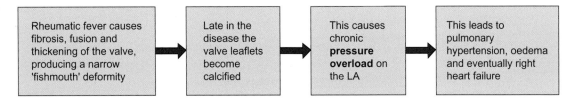

Mitral stenosis typically presents with symptoms of its complications such as **pulmonary oedema**, **RV failure**, **AF** or **thromboembolic phenomena**. The **main risk factor** to elicit is previous **rheumatic fever (24d)**. Remember to exclude other causes of pulmonary hypertension and breathlessness such as COPD and pulmonary embolism.

On peripheral examination, you may find a **malar flush** (cyanotic discoloration of the cheeks) and an irregularly irregular pulse. Palpating the precordium, you may feel a **non-displaced, 'tapping' apex**. The tap represents closure of the stenosed mitral valve (i.e. a palpable S1). **On auscultation**, there is a **loud S1 with or without an opening snap**. The snap represents sudden opening of the mitral valve. In severe mitral stenosis, the snap becomes quieter and moves closer to S2 as the valve is forced to open earlier in diastole by the raised LA pressure **(24e)**. The murmur of mitral stenosis **(24c)** is a **low-pitched mid-diastolic murmur** heard best at the apex with the patient in the left lateral position and is audible with the bell. There may also be a pansystolic murmur of functional tricuspid regurgitation.

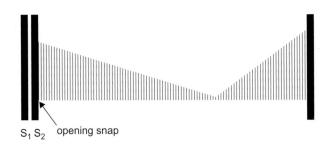

S_1 S_2 opening snap

ECG shows a broad bifid P wave (P mitrale) caused by LA dilatation **(24f)**. A **CXR** may show LA or RV enlargement; signs of LV failure and a lateral view may show a calcified mitral valve. **Echocardiography**: demonstrates valve thickening and reduction in the mid-diastolic closure rate; transoesophageal echocardiography may show visible thrombus in the LA and the Doppler function assesses the pressure gradient across the valve.

Surgery is indicated for refractory dyspnoea or RV failure **(24g)**. **Valvotomy** is performed if the cusps are still pliant and mobile. If they are calcified or incompetent, **valve replacement** is required. **Balloon mitral valvuloplasty** is performed for non-calcified valves, using a transseptal approach from the RA to the LA. This has low morbidity in patients without contraindications. Without surgery, life expectancy is 5–10 years.

Answers

24. a – TB, respiratory neoplasm, chronic bronchitis, heart failure, b – Focal respiratory signs, cardiological signs. Bedside tests: BM stick, dipstick urine, ECG, c–g – See explanation
25. T F (more common in women) T F T
26. F T F T T

27. Regarding tricuspid regurgitation, answer true or false

a. The commonest cause is dilatation of the right ventricle
b. Results in pressure overload of the right ventricle
c. Can be diagnosed by 'end-of-bed inspection' if giant systolic waves of the jugular venous pulse are seen
d. Produces an ejection systolic murmur
e. The murmur is best heard at end-expiration

28. Regarding tricuspid stenosis, answer true or false

a. Is most commonly caused by rheumatoid arthritis
b. Is usually found in association with left heart valve disease
c. Causes pressure overload on the right atrium
d. Produces a mid-diastolic murmur
e. Wide and two-peaked P wave in lead II is the associated electrocardiographic abnormality

29. Regarding pulmonary regurgitation, answer true or false

a. Can be found in association with tetralogy of Fallot
b. Produces volume overload on the right atrium
c. Rapidly causes symptoms of right heart failure
d. Requires urgent surgical treatment
e. Produces a decrescendo early diastolic murmur

30. Regarding pulmonary stenosis, answer true or false

a. Is usually due to a congenital abnormality
b. Causes right ventricular and right atrial hypertrophy
c. Produces a pansystolic murmur
d. Can present with syncope
e. Electrocardiography may show a right ventricular strain pattern

EXPLANATION: RIGHT HEART VALVE DISEASES

Tricuspid regurgitation is usually 'functional' as a result of RV dilatation, however, other causes include **rheumatic fever** and **infective endocarditis**. Tricuspid regurgitation causes **volume overload** of the RV, eventually leading to right heart failure. Patients usually present with **symptoms of right heart failure** such as fatigue, ankle swelling and right upper quadrant pain. Characteristic examination findings include a **pansystolic murmur** heard at the left sternal edge that is loudest in inspiration and associated with an **RV heave**. Peripheral signs include **giant V waves** of the JVP, a **pulsatile, enlarged liver** and **peripheral oedema**. ECG may show **atrial fibrillation** and CXR may show an enlarged heart. **Echocardiography** detects the regurgitant jet, a diseased tricuspid valve and a dilated RV. Management is aimed at treating the underlying cause and reducing symptoms using **ACE inhibitors**, **digoxin** and **diuretics**. **Valve replacement** carries a 20 per cent risk of mortality and is thus reserved for severe cases.

The major cause of **tricuspid stenosis** is **rheumatic fever**, and it is almost always accompanied by mitral or aortic valve disease. It causes **pressure overload** of the RA, raising RA pressure to produce **symptoms of right heart failure**. Examination reveals a **mid-diastolic murmur**, which is low in pitch and heard at the lower left sternal edge, loudest in inspiration. It may be associated with an opening snap. You may also see **giant a waves** of the JVP, representing vigorous RA contraction. The ECG shows **tall-peaked P waves (P pulmonale)**, which are indicative of RA enlargement. CXR is often normal. **Echocardiography** demonstrates a thickened and rigid tricuspid valve associated with RA enlargement. **Valve replacement** is required only in severe cases of right heart failure.

Pulmonary regurgitation can result from any cause of **pulmonary hypertension**. It causes volume overload of the RV, but in most cases is asymptomatic. On examination, you can expect to hear a **decrescendo murmur in early diastole** at the left sternal edge, also known as the **Graham Steell murmur**. ECG may suggest RV hypertrophy and CXR may show enlargement of the RV. **Echocardiography** confirms the valve defect and measures flow across the valve. Treatment is rarely necessary.

Pulmonary stenosis is usually **congenital** and is associated with syndromes such as Turner's syndrome and Tetralogy of Fallot. The stenosis causes **pressure overload** of the RV, resulting in RV hypertrophy. Pulmonary stenosis is often **asymptomatic**, but patients may develop symptoms of reduced pulmonary blood flow such as **fatigue** or **syncope**, or symptoms of **right heart failure**. There is an **ejection systolic murmur** radiating to the left shoulder, loudest at the left sternal edge in inspiration. This may be accompanied by a systolic thrill and an RV heave. ECG may show **right axis deviation**, **P pulmonale** and **right bundle branch block**. On CXR, you may see **post-stenotic dilatation** of the pulmonary artery, **oligaemic lung fields** and **RV/RA hypertrophy**. Echocardiography confirms the valve defect and measures the pressure gradient across the valve. Angiography may be used in children with multiple cardiac abnormalities. **Pulmonary valvotomy** is the mainstay of management.

Answers
27. T F T F F
28. F T T T F
29. F F F F T
30. T T F T T

31. A 76-year-old man is referred to the emergency department by his GP with a four week history of fever, night sweats, anorexia and malaise, following a tooth abscess for which he was seen by his dentist

a. What is your differential diagnosis?
b. What further information would you like to obtain from the history?

When you examine him, you see the following signs: i) splinter haemorrhages, ii) vasculitic rash on limb.

c. What are these signs? What causes them? What are your differential diagnoses now?
d. What other signs would you look for in the examination?
e. On auscultation of the heart, you hear an ejection systolic murmur that radiates to the carotids. What might this represent?

Having examined the patient, you would like to do some investigations.

f. What investigation would you do at the bedside? What would you be looking for and why?
g. What further investigations would you request and why?

Regarding management:

h. What is your immediate management plan?
i. After two weeks, the patient is still complaining of a fever and his C-reactive protein is still raised. What might be the reasons for this lack of improvement in his condition?
j. On auscultation of the heart, you hear a new high-pitched diastolic murmur, loudest at the left sternal edge. What might this represent? What other signs might you expect to elicit?
k. What further management might you consider?
l. What features of this case suggest that the patient may have an adverse prognosis?
m. What further advice would you need to give the patient for the future?

32. What are the known risk factors for infective endocarditis? True or false

a. Bicuspid aortic valve
b. Intravenous drug use
c. Young age
d. Mitral stenosis
e. Patient receiving intravenous cytotoxic chemotherapy
f. Patient with rheumatoid arthritis

EXPLANATION: INFECTIVE ENDOCARDITIS (I)

Infective endocarditis is defined as an infection of the endothelial lining of the heart. **Causative organisms** are divided into those causing **subacute** infection (*Streptococcus viridans* and **enterococci**) and those responsible for **acute** infection (*Streptococcus pneumoniae* and *Staphylococcus aureus*). *S. aureus* causes aggressive valve destruction and is associated with 50 per cent of cases in IV drug users. **Culture-negative endocarditis** is usually the result of partial antibiotic therapy, though some cases may be due to fastidious organisms such as *Chlamydia* or *Coxiella*, or fungal infections such as *Candida* or *Aspergillus*.

Predisposing factors include prosthetic heart valves or structural heart defects (e.g. aortic/mitral valve lesions, ventricular septal defect, patent ductus arteriosus). These cause turbulent blood flow in the heart, which damages the endocardium and promotes formation of avascular platelet–fibrin aggregates or 'vegetations', in which circulating bacteria can become trapped and multiply. IV drug use is associated with right-sided endocarditis, and immunocompromised patients may be susceptible to infection by atypical microorganisms such as fungi.

Endocarditis can present in multiple guises:

- **Sepsis**: Subacute infection presents with fever, night sweats, anorexia and rigors. Acute infection can cause septicaemic shock
- **Valve destruction**: Can cause sudden onset of breathlessness and signs of acute cardiac failure. A **new or changing murmur** is a diagnostic feature **(31d)**
- **Immune complex deposition (31c)** in small vessels can cause **glomerulonephritis**, **arthritis** or **vasculitic lesions** such as splinter haemorrhages (petechial haemorrhages under nails), Janeway lesions (non-tender red lesions on palms), Osler's nodes (tender red nodules on finger pulps), petechial/purpuric skin rash and Roth spots in the eye
- **Chronic infection**: causes clubbing, anaemia and splenomegaly **(31d)**
- **Septic embolization**: to major organs or extremities can cause septic abscesses and persisting fever **(31d)**
- **Direct extension of vegetations**: can cause conduction defects, valve ring abscesses or mycotic aneuryms.

Differential diagnoses to consider when assessing patients presenting with symptoms and signs of endocarditis **(31a)** include meningococcal septicaemia (ask about photophobia and neck stiffness), viral illness, hidden abscesses, TB, lymphoma, rheumatic heart disease and inflammatory vasculitic conditions **(31c)** (e.g. SLE, rheumatoid arthritis).

Answers

31. a – See explanation, b – Risk factors for infective endocarditis, c–d – See explanation, e – Aortic stenosis, f – Urinalysis: haematuria and proteinuria due to glomerulonephritis, g–i – See explanation on page 97, j – Aortic regurgitation due to aortic valve destruction. Other signs: collapsing pulse, wide pulse pressure, displaced apex beat, k – Surgical intervention, l – Aortic valve involvement, m – Antibiotic prophylaxis
32. T T F T F F

33. How should blood cultures be taken in patients with suspected infective endocarditis? True or false

    a. One anaerobic bottle and one aerobic bottle from the antecubital fossa
    b. Two aerobic bottles and one anaerobic bottle from the antecubital fossa
    c. Three samples of two bottles over three weeks from three different sites
    d. Three samples of two bottles from the same site more than 12 hours apart
    e. Three samples of two bottles from three different sites less than 12 hours apart
    f. Fill the aerobic bottle before you fill the anaerobic bottle

34. Regarding pathogens in infective endocarditis (true or false?)

    a. *Staphylococcus aureus* is the most common causative pathogen
    b. *Staphylococcus aureus* valve infection typically presents in an insidious manner
    c. *Streptococcus viridans* infection is associated with dental treatment
    d. Candidal infection may produce culture-negative endocarditis
    e. The most common pathogen in intravenous drug users is *Streptococcus pneumoniae*

35. Which of the following patients fulfil the Duke criteria for the diagnosis of infective endocarditis?

    a. A patient with three sets of blood cultures positive for *Staphylococcus aureus* and a new diastolic murmur heard loudest at the left sternal edge with the patient leaning forwards in end-expiration
    b. An intravenous drug user who is pyrexial (38.9°C) with three sets of blood cultures positive for *Staphylococcus aureus*
    c. An elderly woman with a pre-existing ejection systolic murmur, splinter haemorrhages and mild splenomegaly in whom echocardiography shows a large vegetation on the aortic valve

36. Regarding treatment of infective endocarditis, answer true or false

    a. Never wait for the results of the blood cultures before starting antibiotic therapy
    b. Surgical replacement of the valve is indicated in all cases of endocarditis
    c. Liaise early with the microbiological team in cases of infective endocarditis
    d. Most patients with prosthetic heart valves do not require antibiotic prophylaxis before dental surgery

CRP, C-reactive protein

EXPLANATION: INFECTIVE ENDOCARDITIS (II)

Infective endocarditis is diagnosed according to the **Duke criteria** (two major criteria *or* one major and three minor criteria *or* five minor criteria), which require two **investigations (31g)**:

- **Blood cultures**: Three sets of two bottles (aerobic and anaerobic) are taken from three separate sites at different times. If clinical conditions permit, take samples more than 12 hours apart before starting antibiotic therapy. The blood cultures are the only investigation that can accurately guide which antibiotics should be used
- **Echocardiography**: Visualizes large vegetations and detects underlying valvular disease or resultant valvular regurgitation or abscesses. **Transoesophageal echocardiography** is more sensitive than transthoracic echocardiography.

Major criteria	Minor criteria
Persistently positive blood cultures	Risk factors for endocarditis
Endocardial involvement (new or changing murmur or echocardiographic evidence)	Fever >38°C
	Vascular complications
	Immunological complications
	Suggestive blood cultures (not meeting major criteria)
	Suggestive echocardiography (not meeting major criteria)

FBC may show neutrophilia and **normochromic normocytic anaemia**. **CRP** and **ESR** are usually raised. Check for haematuria, red cell casts and proteinuria in the urine, and measure serum **urea** and **creatinine** to exclude glomerulonephritis.

Initial management **(31h)** is **IV antibiotic therapy**. Ideally, await blood culture positivity before starting antibiotics, but if sepsis is too severe to permit delay, take a large number of blood cultures then start an empirical regimen such as benzylpenicillin and gentamicin. In acute cases, add flucloxacillin to cover staphylococci. Liaise early and remain in contact with microbiology. Combination therapy is usually continued for two weeks and monotherapy for a further two to four weeks for prosthetic valves. For persisting/recurring fever, consider changing the antibiotics or adding antifungals (e.g. amphotericin). **Persisting fever** may indicate **immune complex deposition or abscess formation (31i)**. **Valve replacement** is indicated for prosthetic valve infection, significant valvular regurgitation, infection with *S. aureus* (valve destruction), fungal infection (drugs are fungistatic, not fungicidal), conduction defects, abscess formation, recurrent embolism or large, resistant infections.

In most cases, the fever and systemic upset resolve within one week of starting antibiotics. The **overall mortality is 15–30 per cent**. An adverse prognosis is associated with infection with *Staphylococcus* or enterococci, culture-negative endocarditis, aortic valve involvement, and renal or cerebral complications. **Antibiotic prophylaxis** before dental treatment or upper respiratory tract, genitourinary or gastrointestinal procedures is required in patients with prosthetic valves and in those who have had a previous episode of infective endocarditis.

Answers

33. F F F F F F (fill anaerobic bottle first to prevent any air in syringe entering bottle)
34. T F T T F
35. T F T
36. F F T F

37. A 57-year-old woman presents with a 2-day history of chest pain and feeling unwell. She tells you that the pain came on gradually over the last 2 days. It is not related to exertion or to food. She feels feverish and has been breathless today

    a. What is your differential diagnosis?
    b. What features of the chest pain would make you think of pericarditis?
    c. What signs would you specifically look for in the examination?

On examination, she looks unwell. She is sitting forwards in her bed and is breathless on speaking. Her heart rate is 120 bpm, her BP 140/70 mmHg, her temperature 38.1°C, her respiratory rate 18 breaths per minute and her oxygen saturation 94 per cent on air. You notice that her hands are deformed, with ulnar deviation at the metacarpophalangeal joints. On auscultation of the heart, you hear a scratching sound throughout the cardiac cycle.

    d. What features of the history and examination worry you most?
    e. What might be the significance of the hand deformity?
    f. What initial investigation would you request?
    g. The electrocardiogram looks like this. What is the major abnormality?

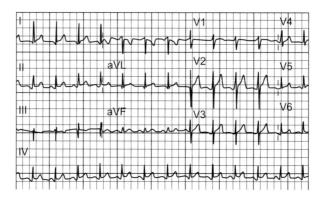

    h. What is your management plan?

38. Regarding pericardial tamponade, answer true or false

    a. Tamponade occurs when the intrapericardial pressure equals or exceeds the intraventricular pressure, preventing ventricular filling in diastole
    b. Tamponade is a medical emergency
    c. Chest radiography shows a small heart
    d. Echocardiography demonstrates impaired diastolic filling and an echo-free area around the heart

S3, third heart sound; ZN, Ziehl–Neelsen

EXPLANATION: PERICARDIAL DISEASE

Causes of **acute pericarditis** (inflammation of the pericardium) include **infection** (coxsackievirus, TB, pneumonia), **recent MI** (Dressler's syndrome), **inflammatory conditions** (rheumatoid disease **(37e)**, SLE) and **uraemia**, or it can be **idiopathic**. Acute pericarditis presents with central or left-sided **chest pain** that is sharp and persistent in nature, radiates to the neck or shoulders and is relieved by sitting forwards **(37b)**. There are **systemic symptoms** of fever, malaise and arthralgia. On examination, you will hear a **pericardial friction rub**, a high-pitched scratch throughout the cardiac cycle that changes with position **(37c)**. The **ECG (37f)** characteristically shows concave or 'saddle-shaped' ST elevation in all leads **(31g)**, though in 10 per cent of cases it is normal or shows non-specific changes. Treatment **(37h)** is symptomatic with **NSAIDs**, and the illness should resolve spontaneously in one to two weeks. Relapse or persistent inflammation is treated with **colchicines, corticosteroids** or **immunosuppressants**. It is important to address and treat the **underlying cause**.

Constrictive pericarditis (fibrotic thickening of the pericardial sac) restricts diastolic filling. It may result from recurrent pericarditis (15–40 per cent of acute pericarditis), TB, malignant infiltrations or radiotherapy. The symptoms are those of **raised atrial pressure** such as dyspnoea, reduced exercise tolerance and abdominal discomfort. On examination, the **JVP is raised** with rapid x and y descent and there is a **positive Kussmaul's sign** (increased engorgement of neck veins on inspiration). The **apex beat is soft and diffuse**, **heart sounds are quiet** and a **diastolic pericardial knock** (filling sound) may be heard before S3. ECG usually shows non-specific changes such as atrial fibrillation or ST segment abnormalities and CXR shows a small heart, sometimes with pericardial calcification. **Echocardiography** shows **abnormal diastolic function** and **cardiac catheterization** shows **equal pressures** in the four cardiac chambers. **Surgical resection** of the parietal pericardium is required to prevent progression; however, short-term palliation can be achieved with diuretics.

Pericardial effusion is accumulation of fluid in the pericardial sac as a result of inflammation of the parietal pericardium. This may not become clinically apparent until the fluid volume increases enough to cause **dyspnoea**, **reduced exercise tolerance** and **engorgement of the neck veins**. Other signs include **tachypnoea, tachycardia, pulsus paradoxus** (exaggerated reduction in systolic BP on inspiration), **raised JVP** (with exaggerated x descent and no y descent), bronchial breathing at the left lung base (due to compression of the left lower lobe, **Ewart's sign**) and **quiet heart sounds**. ECG shows **low-voltage complexes** and **electrical alternans** of the QRS complex (reflecting beat-to-beat variation in ventricular filling). CXR shows an **enlarged, globular heart** and on echocardiography there is a dark, **echo-free zone** around the heart. **Pericardiocentesis** is used for diagnosis and therapy. The fluid drained should be sent for culture, ZN staining and cytology. **Recurrent effusions**, such as malignant effusions, can be treated surgically by creating a window between the pericardial and pleural/abdominal space.

Pericardial tamponade is defined as pericardial fluid accumulation such that the intrapericardial pressure exceeds the ventricular diastolic pressure, leading to impaired ventricular filling and reduced cardiac output. In the acute setting, it is usually caused by haemorrhage. The symptoms are similar to those of severe pericardial effusion and depend on the rapidity of fluid development. Look for **Beck's triad: 1) falling BP, 2) rising JVP and 3) quiet heart sounds**. Seek specialist help as the effusion should be drained urgently and the fluid sent to the laboratory for culture, ZN stain and cytology. It is essential to address the underlying cause.

Answers

37. a – Aortic dissection, acute coronary syndrome, angina, respiratory causes, b–c – See explanation, d – Pericardial friction rub with dyspnoea, tachycardia and tachypnoea: suggests pericardial effusion, e–h – See explanation
38. T T F (enlarged, globular heart) T T

39. You are working in the developing world when a 10-year-old child is brought to you by his mother. You gather that he had a sore throat for a few days last week and has been complaining of pain in his knee and shoulder. His mother has noticed a rash on his abdomen. On examination, his heart rate is 160 bpm and his temperature is 39.2°C. You hear a pansystolic murmur radiating to the axilla. On his trunk, you see a red rash with a raised edge and white centre

    a. What is the diagnosis?
    b. What are the criteria for diagnosing this condition? Does this child fit the criteria?
    c. What investigations would you like to do?
    d. How would you treat this child?
    e. There are no antibiotics available in the region. What is this child's risk of death?

40. **Regarding the pathophysiology of rheumatic fever, answer true or false**

    a. Rheumatic fever is the result of an immune response to group B *Streptococcus* antigens
    b. Streptococcal protein antigens mimic cellular proteins on cardiac valves
    c. The antibodies produced in rheumatic fever can affect the lungs, joints and central nervous system
    d. Socio-economic conditions play a role in determining the risk of developing rheumatic heart disease
    e. The Aschoff body is a pathognomonic lesion found in rheumatic fever

41. **Which of the following cases can be diagnosed as rheumatic fever?**

    a. A patient with no history of a sore throat but arthritis and a red, migrating rash
    b. A patient with raised antistreptolysin-O titres, raised erythrocyte sedimentation rate and arthralgia
    c. A patient with a positive throat swab, a heart murmur and unilateral involuntary movements

42. **Regarding the management of rheumatic fever, answer true or false**

    a. Patients should be allowed to mobilize as soon as they feel better
    b. Corticosteroids are important in preventing recurrence of the disease
    c. Non-steroidal anti-inflammatory drugs should be given for carditis and arthritis
    d. Prophylactic antibiotics should be continued for 5 years

ASO, antistreptolysin-O; CRP, C-reactive protein

EXPLANATION: RHEUMATIC FEVER

Worldwide, rheumatic fever accounts for 25–50 per cent of all cardiac hospital admissions, though in the West the incidence has decreased significantly over the last 30 years. It is an **immunological sequela** to pharyngeal infection with **Lancefield group A haemolytic streptococci**. Antibodies to carbohydrate antigens cross-react with cardiac valve tissue, causing pancarditis. The antibodies also affect the joints, lungs and CNS. Susceptibility to cardiac damage is influenced by age, socio-economic conditions, ethnicity, genetic factors and climate.

Rheumatic fever is diagnosed using the **revised Jones criteria (39b)**, which require evidence of recent streptococcal infection plus two major criteria or one major plus two minor criteria **(39c)**.

Evidence of streptococcal infection	Major criteria	Minor criteria
Recently diagnosed streptococcal infection	**Carditis**: tachycardia, new regurgitant murmur, pericardial rub, signs of cardiac failure, conduction defects	Fever
History of scarlet fever	**Arthritis**: migratory, large joints	Raised ESR/CRP
Positive throat swab	**Skin**: painless, mobile **nodules** on extensor surfaces, **erythema marginatum** (red raised rash with clear centre) on trunk, thighs, arms	Arthralgia
Increase in ASO titre		Prolonged PR interval
Increase in DNase B titre	**CNS**: Sydenham's chorea: occurs late in disease, involuntary unilateral movements, associated with emotional and behavioural lability	Previous rheumatic fever

Management (39d) relies on **antibiotics** such as benzylpenicillin or penicillin V and **bed rest** util the CRP has been normal for two weeks. Carditis and arthritis can be treated symptomatically with **NSAIDs**. Corticosteroids may improve symptoms but do not affect prognosis. Chorea is treated with haloperidol. **Antibiotic prophylaxis** is continued for 5 years after an acute attack, as it has been shown to reduce late mortality and prevent recurrent infection.

On average, acute attacks last for **three months**. **Recurrence** can be triggered by another streptococcal infection, pregnancy or the oral contraceptive pill. Sixty per cent of patients with carditis go on to develop chronic **rheumatic heart disease**, affecting the mitral valve in 70 per cent and the aortic valve in 40 per cent. **Incompetent valves** may develop **during** the attack, whereas **stenosed valves** may develop **years later**. Untreated, mortality from rheumatic fever is 25 per cent **(39e)**; this is reduced to 1 per cent with antibiotic therapy.

Answers

39. a – Rheumatic fever, b–e – See explanation
40. F (group A) F (carbohydrate antigens, not protein antigens) T T T
41. c
42. F F T T

43. Concerning essential/primary hypertension (true or false)

   a. It accounts for 90–95 per cent of patients and has an easily identifiable cause
   b. It occurs in individuals under 30 years causing hypokalaemia and renal dysfunction
   c. It is more resistant to treatment than secondary hypertension
   d. High salt intake, smoking, alcohol and obesity are all protective factors

44. The following are causes of secondary hypertension, true or false

   a. Glomerulonephritis
   b. Addison's disease
   c. Hypopituitarism
   d. Phaeochromocytoma
   e. Oestrogens

45. What are the long-term risks and effects of hypertension?

46. Place the following effects of hypertension on the retina in order of increasing severity from grade 1 to 4

   a. Flame haemorrhages and cotton wool spots
   b. Papilloedema
   c. Nipping of the venules at arteriovenous crossings
   d. Increased tortuosity of retinal vessels and increased reflectiveness (silver-wiring appearance)

47. When choosing treatment for a patient with hypertension, you might preferentially prescribe (true or false)

   a. An angiotensin-converting enzyme inhibitor for a patient with left ventricular failure
   b. A beta-blocker for a patient with a history of asthma
   c. Diltiazem with a beta-blocker

EXPLANATION: CHRONIC HYPERTENSION

Hypertension is any BP greater than 140 mmHg systolic over 90 mmHg diastolic. Roughly one-third of the hypertensive population are unaware that they have high BP. This is mainly because 90–95 per cent have **essential hypertension**; that is, without an obvious cause or prominent symptoms.

The Framingham heart study concluded that systolic BP is the most important determinant of cardiovascular risk in patients over 50 years old **(46)**. To reduce this risk, national guidelines have been introduced to screen for hypertension in the community. Because BP can increase in clinical settings and vary with the time of day, three readings are recommended before a diagnosis is made or treatment commenced.

Young age, resistance to treatment, renal dysfunction and hypokalaemia are features suggestive of secondary hypertension. The main causes of secondary hypertensions can be considered as **renal** (e.g. renal artery stenosis, chronic glomerulonephritis, polyarteritis nodosa, polycystic kidney disease, chronic pyelonephritis and systemic sclerosis), or **endocrine** (e.g. phaeochromocytoma, Cushing's syndrome, Conn's syndrome, acromegaly, polycystic ovary syndrome and hyperparathyroidism).

Once hypertension has been diagnosed, there are three important tasks: 1) exclude secondary causes, 2) look for end-organ damage, as this indicates the duration, severity and prognosis and 3) assess the risk of cardiovascular disease, as this may impact on management.

LV hypertrophy is a compensatory response to chronically elevated BP that can be detected on examination and confirmed by ECG or echocardiography. Renovascular damage and glomerular loss resulting from hypertension can be detected by dipstick for proteinurea, blood tests for U&Es or renal ultrasonography. Fundoscopy should be performed and the stage of hypertensive retinopathy recorded **(45)**.

Lifestyle changes such as a careful diet (low salt, low fat and plenty of fruit and vegetables) and exercise have been shown to reduce BP. Drug treatment is divided into four main classes: **A** – ACE inhibitors and angiotensin II antagonists; **B** – beta-blockers (no longer preferred as routine first-line therapy for hypertension: *J Hypertens* 2006;**24**:2131–41); **C** – calcium channel antagonists; **D** – diuretics. These drugs are discussed in more detail on page 123, but there are a few useful tips (see www.nice.org.UK/guidance/CG34/guidance/pdf/English for more details):

- Most drugs take four to eight weeks to take full effect
- Beta-blockers are no longer recommended as routine initial therapy for hypertension, but can be considered in young people; for example, women of childbearing age, patients with evidence of increased sympathetic tone and those with contraindications to ACE inhibitors or angiotensin II antagonists
- If a patient using a beta-blocker requires a second antihypertensive medication, choose a calcium channel blocker rather than a thiazide diuretic to reduce the patient's risk of developing diabetes.

Answers
43. F F F F
44. T F F T T
45. See explanation
46. d, c, a, b
47. T F (contraindicated)   F (dangerous and may cause severe bradycardia)

A 39-year-old Afro-Carribean female teacher presents to A&E with a 2-day history of increasingly severe headache and 2 hours of blurred vision and vomiting. The headache has increased gradually over the last 2 days, her vision has been slightly blurred and 2 hours ago she started vomiting. You take her BP and it is 225/130 mmHg.

48. What is the likely diagnosis?

49. True or false?

   a. Malignant or accelerated hypertension usually occurs on a background of essential hypertension
   b. Accelerated hypertension is characterized by papilloedema
   c. Renal artery stenosis is a side effect of malignant or accelerated hypertension
   d. Untreated, the 1-year survival rate is around 90 per cent
   e. Angiotensin-converting enzyme inhibitors should initially be avoided because of the risk of renal decompensation
   f. Blood pressure needs to be brought down to within the normal range in the first hour

You go in search of an ophthalmoscope, and when you return to perform fundoscopy you notice that she is drowsy. You wake her up and she seems slightly confused. On examining the fundus, you see small haemorrhages and the optic disc looks swollen.

50. What complication may have developed? Name two other dangerous complications

51. From the following list of investigations, decide what each might show and state whether it is related to cause or effect

   a. Electrocardiography
   b. Urea and electrolytes and creatinine
   c. Urine microscopy
   d. Renal ultrasonography
   e. Pregnancy test

52. Which two of the following treatments would be least appropriate in her initial treatment?

   a. Intravenous infusion of glyceryl trinitrate
   b. Intravenous labetolol
   c. Oral amlodipine
   d. Sublingual nifedipine
   e. Oral frusemide

EXPLANATION: MALIGNANT OR ACCELERATED HYPERTENSION

Accelerated hypertension is severe uncontrolled hypertension, with BP often exceeding 220/120 mmHg and retinal changes such as haemorrhages or exudates. Malignant hypertension is characterized by papilloedema. Both present due to an acute rise in BP with symptoms including headaches, confusion and visual disturbance.

The commonest cause is acute exacerbation of essential hypertension, but it can occur secondary to pregnancy, renal artery stenosis, acute food reaction while taking a monoamine oxidase inhibitor, phaeochromocytoma or pregnancy. Dangerous complications are heart failure, renal failure and encephalopathy **(50)**.

Management is controlled reduction in BP over days rather than hours. Even with symptoms of encephalopathy, diastolic BP should be brought down to a target of 110 mmHg over 4–6 hours. Aggressive BP reduction carries a risk of stroke and tissue ischaemia, as the tissues have adapted to require a high perfusion pressure and take time to return to normal when the pressures are reduced by medication.

The drugs indicated are frusemide (IV or oral), which can be supplemented with a thiazide diuretic, beta-blockers or a long-acting calcium channel antagonist. Sublingual nifedipine can cause an uncontrollable drop in BP and is therefore particularly dangerous in this situation **(52)**. GTN is a relatively weak arteriolar dilator and should not be used as first-line therapy **(52)**.

Malignant or accelerated hypertension is very dangerous, and the prognosis is poor if it is untreated; up to 90 per cent of cases die in within 1 year, usually from end-organ damage and failure.

Answers

48. Malignant or accelerated hypertension
49. T F F F T F
50. Encephalopathy; heart failure, renal failure; see explanation
51. a – LV hypertrophy (background of chronic hypertension), MI (effect), b – Hypokalaemia – phaeochromocytoma (cause), renal failure (effect), c – Glomerulonephritis (cause), renal damage (effect), d – Small kidney – renal artery stenosis (cause), e – Pregnancy (cause)
52. a, d. See explanation

Mrs S is a 73-year-old woman who presented to her GP with a four-week history of becoming increasingly breathless and easily fatigued by mild activities such as getting dressed or cooking. She has had a reduced appetite for about two weeks. Her past medical history includes mild asthma, which is well controlled with an inhaler. She is a lifelong non-smoker and takes no other regular medication.

53. What is your differential diagnosis?

The GP examined her and noticed that she was tachycardic with a raised JVP, ankle oedema and a 2 cm smooth liver edge.

54. Which of the following are causes of a raised JVP?

a. Fluid overload
b. Bicuspid aortic valve
c. Right heart failure
d. Atrioventricular block
e. Superior vena cava obstruction

55. Of the following causes of heart failure (i) which one is most common and (ii) would you associate them with right heart failure, left heart failure or both?

a. Pulmonary embolism
b. Myocardial infarction
c. Atrial septal defect
d. Cardiomyopathy
e. Pericardial constriction

56. You decide that she is in right heart failure. Given that moderate physical activity has made her breathless and easily fatigued

a. How would you classify this on the New York Heart association scale (I–IV)?
b. What investigations would you want to perform?
c. What treatment would you recommend if heart failure is confirmed?
d. What medication would you not give her and why?

LVH, left ventricular hypertrophy

EXPLANATION: CHRONIC HEART FAILURE

Heart failure is an inability to maintain sufficient cardiac output to adequately perfuse the body. It can be characterized as right heart failure, left heart failure or a combination of the two, **congestive cardiac failure**. **Right heart failure** is usually a chronic process with a slow onset of symptoms that are caused by congestion of the peripheral circulation. **Left heart failure** can present insidiously or acutely, if decompensation occurs, with sudden failure to maintain cardiac output. Most cases of heart failure are a combination of left- and right-sided dysfunction, but the pathology and symptoms may be attributable more to one side than the other.

Clinically the most useful classification is by **cause**. The most common cause is **MI**, which accounts for more than half of all cases of heart failure in the UK. Other common causes include LVH and cardiomyopathy. By considering the heart in its role as a pump, the causes of heart failure can be classified according to the way that they lead to inadequate function:

- Inadequate filling – mitral stenosis, LVH, pericardial constriction
- Inadequate pump force generation – MI, muscle damage, cardiomyopathy, myocarditis
- Volume overload – fluid overload (iatrogenic), aortic or mitral regurgitation
- Increased resistance – aortic or pulmonary stenosis, systemic or pulmonary hypertension
- Increased demand (high-output states) – anaemia, thyrotoxicosis, beriberi

Causes more specific to right heart failure include chronic pulmonary hypertension, cor pulmonale, pulmonary embolism, tricuspid or pulmonary valve damage and ventricular septal defect.

Right heart failure
Elevated JVP
Hepatomegaly
Peripheral oedema
Dyspnoea
Pulsatile liver
Ascites

Left heart failure
Dyspnoea
Paroxysmal nocturnal dyspnoea
Tachycardia
Tachypnoea
Basal crepitations

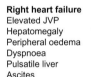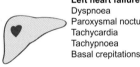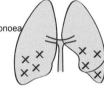

Investigations for heart failure
Echocardiography, ECG – damaged valves, MI, LVH
CXR – Kerley B lines, enlarged heart
Cardiac catheterization
Bloods, full blood count, thyroid function tests etc.

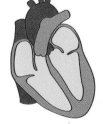

Treatment for heart failure
Prognostic   ACE inhibitors or angiotensin II
           Beta-blockers (CIBIS II trial)
           Spironolactone (RALES trial)
           Exercise rehabilitation (ExTraMatch)
Palliative   Fluid restriction, low-salt diet
           Diuretics
           Digoxin

Careful assessment of fluid balance and daily weights are an important part of the management of patients with heart failure. The prognosis is poor; only one-fifth of patients survive more than 5 years after diagnosis.

Answers

53. Right heart failure and/or left heart failure, heart block, anaemia, pneumonia, aortic stenosis
54. a, c, e
55. (i) b; (ii) a – right, b – both, c – right, d – both, e – both
56. a – III, b – ECG, echocardiography, CXR, c – ACE inhibitors, diuretics to palliate oedema, advice on diet and exercise, d – Beta-blocker, due to pre-existing asthma

A 52-year-old man presents to A&E. He is extremely short of breath and his ankles are swollen. He has a 4-day history of increasing shortness of breath, he has not been able to sleep lying down for the last two nights because it feels like he is drowning, and he has presented to A&E because this morning he started coughing up 'pink froth'.

---

57. (a) What is your differential diagnosis? (b) What is your immediate management?

On examination, he is pale and sweaty, though afebrile. His pulse is 170 bpm and irregular, his JVP is raised to 4 cm, his blood pressure is 130/80 mmHg and he has marked ankle oedema and crackles at both lung bases.

---

58. Causes of acute heart failure include (true or false)

    a. Myocardial infarction
    b. Sudden-onset arrhythmias such as atrial fibrillation
    c. Endocarditis
    d. Ventricular septal defect
    e. Phaeochromocytoma

---

59. For the following possible diagnoses in this patient, choose the most appropriate investigation and think about the findings that you would expect. You may choose more than one investigation

Options

    A. Arrhythmia due to hyperkalaemia   **C.** Valve chordal rupture
    B. Myocarditis   **D.** Myocardial infarction

    1. Full blood count
    2. Urea and electrolytes
    3. Blood cultures
    4. Viral serology
    5. Biomarkers such as troponin
    6. Electrocardiography
    7. Chest radiography
    8. Echocardiography
    9. Right heart catheterization

COPD, chronic obstructive pulmonary disease; CPAP, continuous positive airway pressure

EXPLANATION: ACUTE HEART FAILURE

Heart failure can present acutely in two main situations: (a) an **acute event** has caused a normally healthy individual to develop heart failure or (b) a patient already in **chronic** heart failure that is normally well controlled suddenly **decompensates**.

Causes of (a) include **acute MI**, myocarditis, acute damage to valves (endocarditis, tear or chordal rupture), acute ventricular septal defect, acute hypertensive crisis (malignant hypertension, renal artery stenosis, phaeochromocytoma), severe bradycardia or tachycardia, cardiac tamponade and toxic levels of drugs. Causes of (b) include **non-compliance** with heart failure medication, other **illness** (e.g. pneumonia, anaemia, thyrotoxicosis) or volume load putting extra strain on the heart, MI and arrhythmias.

Management of acute heart failure includes the following steps **(57b)**:

- Resuscitate (ABC), sit up, give **oxygen**
- IV **furosemide** 40–80 mg bolus
- IV **diamorphine** 2.5–5.0 mg plus metoclopramide 10 mg
- Sublingual GTN, or an infusion of intravenous nitrates can be titrated to maintain a low systolic BP (<100 mmHg)
- Consider: LMWH anticoagulation if in atrial fibrillation, aspirin if suggestion of ischaemia.

Monitoring and subsequent management may include transfer to ICU and includes:

- Heart rate, BP, continuous heart rhythm, oxygen saturation
- When obtaining IV access, take bloods: FBC (anaemia) U&Es, Mg^{2+}, glucose, thyroid-stimulating hormone, liver functions tests, cardiac enzymes
- Arterial blood gas (especially if COPD)
- Catheterize; ensure urine output >30 mL/hour
- Consider a central line and inotropes if in cardiogenic shock
- Consider an arterial line if CPAP or ventilation is needed for resistant hypoxia.

Complications of heart failure include:

- **Renal failure**: in the acute setting, diuresis may be insufficient to combat extreme fluid overload, and in extreme cases venesection has been used
- **Respiratory failure**: hypoxia, hypercapnia and acidosis may result in an exhausted patient in respiratory compromise; this situation is unlikely to be reversed without ventilation or CPAP
- **Ventricular arrhythmias**: these can lead to sudden death and contribute to almost half of deaths due to chronic heart failure; syncope may also be a resultant feature
- **Atrial fibrillation**: can be both the cause and a consequence of heart failure; manage with warfarin plus a beta-blocker or digoxin for rate control or DC cardioversion to restore rhythm
- **Thromboembolism**: the high risk of arrhythmias goes hand-in-hand with a high risk of systemic emboli; elderly, immobile patients also have a high risk of DVT or pulmonary embolism; LMWH or warfarin prophylaxis may be indicated.

Answers

57. a – Acute heart failure, pneumonia, acute respiratory distress syndrome, pulmonary oedema, asthma/COPD, b – See explanation
58. T T T T T
59. A – 2 (high K^+), – 6 (atrial fibrillation and tenting of T waves); B – 3 (may show meningococcus, clostridia, diptheria), – 4 (may indicate coxsackievirus, polio, HIV), – 6 (atrioventricular block, ST segment elevation or depression, T wave inversion); C – 6 (changes), – 8 (chordal rupture); D – 5 (troponin elevated days after MI), – 7 (ST changes or pathological Q waves)

60. An ASD (true or false)

a. Is acquired over time
b. Allows blood to shunt from left to right
c. Causes an aortic ejection systolic murmur
d. May be associated with atrial fibrillation
e. Can lead to Eisenmenger's syndrome

61. Choose from the following list of symptoms and signs which ones are most likely to be associated with an ASD

a. Dyspnoea
b. Splinter haemorrhages
c. Fatigue
d. Cyanosis
e. Head nodding

62. Attribute the following possible ASD features to primum, secundum or both

a. Electrocardiographic changes may show right bundle branch block
b. Electrocardiographic changes may show right ventricular hypertrophy
c. Electrocardiographic changes may show right axis deviation
d. Often involves the atrioventricular valves
e. May present later in life with symptoms of heart failure
f. Risk of endocarditis is significant

63. Concerning investigations and treatment of ASD (true or false)

a. Electrocardiography is diagnostic
b. Surgical closure is recommended only over the age of 40 years
c. Cardiac catheterization shows that oxygen saturation in the right atrium is normal
d. In secundum, percutaneous closure techniques may avoid the need for surgery
e. There is no medical treatment

ASD, atrial septal defect; S2, second heart sound

EXPLANATION: CONGENITAL CARDIAC DISEASE: ATRIAL SEPTAL DEFECT

An ASD is a congenital opening between the RA and LA. When pulmonary vascular resistance decreases shortly after birth, oxygenated blood is shunted from left to right. This causes an increase in RA and RV load leading to right heart dilatation, an increase in pulmonary blood flow and a resulting increase in the size of the pulmonary arteries and veins.

The defect can usually be identified as either primum or secundum. **Secundum** is the most common, accounting for around 70 per cent of defects. It is less severe and often does not present until adulthood, when an individual aged 40–60 years has shortness of breath on exertion, fatigue and symptoms of heart failure. **Primum** often involves the atrioventricular valves and therefore can lead to mitral or tricuspid regurgitation. This usually presents in childhood with breathlessness and cyanosis. Median life expectancy with a defect that is not repaired operatively is 30 years. Supraventricular tachycardias such as atrial fibrillation can also be associated with an ASD.

Examination may reveal an irregularly irregular heartbeat, raised JVP, wide fixed splitting of S2 and an ejection systolic murmur. There may be peripheral oedema or crackles at the lung bases.

The investigation of choice is **echocardiography**, as this is diagnostic **(63a)**. ECG features include right bundle branch block and RV hypetrophy. Primum is commonly associated with left axis deviation, while secundum often leads to right axis deviation. A prolonged PR interval may also occur with a primum defect. CXR features can include atrial enlargement and a small aortic knuckle. Cardiac catheterization invariably shows increased oxygen saturation in the RA.

In children, surgical closure is recommended, especially in those with a primum defect presenting before the age of 10 years. Repair or replacement of the mitral valve may be required when patch-closing a primum defect. The role of surgery in an older patient is controversial, as the risks of cardiac failure and cerebral embolism are much greater. In secundum, percutaneous closure may be possible. Although there is no medical cure for ASD, pharmacological control of symptoms has been shown to be beneficial for those in heart failure and can lead to a dramatic improvement in their quality of life.

Answers
60. F T F T T
61. a, c, d
62. both, both, secundum, primum, secundum, primum
63. F F F T F

64. Which of the presentations below may be due to a VSD? (true or false)

a. An infant with heart failure
b. An adolescent with breathlessness, fatigue and cyanosis
c. An adult with effort syncope, clubbing and heart failure
d. Detected incidentally as a murmur during a routine health check

65. Eisenmenger's syndrome may result from pulmonary hypertension occurring in addition to (true or false)

a. An atrial septal defect
b. A ventricular septal defect
c. Mitral stenosis
d. Aortic regurgitation
e. Patent ductus arteriosus

66. Choose from the list below the one best option for the short-term and long-term treatment of these three conditions

Options

A. Heart-lung transplant
B. Banding the pulmonary artery forming a stenosis
C. Ventricular septal defect repair
D. Medical treatment
E. Bypassing the pulmonary artery stenosis with a graft/shunt

1. Ventricular septal defect
2. Eisenmenger's complex
3. Tetralogy of Fallot

VSD, ventricular septal defect; LVH, left ventricular hypertrophy; RVH, right ventricular hypertrophy

EXPLANATION: CONGENITAL CARDIAC DISEASE: VENTRICULAR SEPTAL DEFECT, EISENMENGER'S SYNDROME AND TETRALOGY OF FALLOT

VSD is the most common **congenital** heart defect; 1 in every 500 babies are born with a hole in the septum between their ventricles. Some remain asymptomatic and others recover completely; 40 per cent of defects are believed to close during childhood. A VSD may also be **acquired**; for example, due to an MI.

The symptoms, signs and management of VSD vary with the size and site of the defect.

Small VSDs may be asymptomatic. Examination findings include a systolic thrill, a left parasternal heave and a loud murmur. ECG and CXR are usually normal. Some small VSDs close spontaneously and thus do not require any surgical intervention. **Moderate-size VSDs** may present in adolescence or in later life. The examination findings are similar to those with small VSDs, but ECG may show left axis deviation and LVH, and there may be pulmonary plethora on CXR. **Large VSDs** present with severe heart failure at the age of two to four months, but the murmur is quiet. ECG shows both LVH and RVH, and CXR shows a large heart and prominent pulmonary vessels. Large or symptomatic shunts should be closed surgically.

If a moderate or large congenital VSD is detected early, **artificial stenosis** of the pulmonary arteries can be performed by banding them **(66)**. This protects the pulmonary system from the high pressures created on the right side of the heart. The VSD can then be repaired at a later stage **(66)**. VSD should not be dealt with surgically if pulmonary hypertension has already developed, as this leads to a reversal in the direction of the shunt from right to left, leading to **Eisenmenger's syndrome**.

Eisenmenger's syndrome is the right to left shunting of deoxygenated blood through an ASD, patent ductus arteriosus or VSD due to **pulmonary hypertension**. Symptoms include dyspnoea, central and peripheral cyanosis, haemoptysis, angina and exertional syncope. Pharmacological treatment or venesection may reduce these symptoms **(66)**, though in most cases the only cure is **heart and lung transplantation (66)**. The average life expectancy after such a procedure is relatively low at 7 years.

Tetralogy of Fallot represents approximately 10 per cent of cases of congenital cardiac disease and is one of the causes of a **blue baby**. The baby is born with a combination of four defects that alter the direction of flow through the heart. These are 1) a **VSD**, 2) an **overriding aorta**, 3) **pulmonary stenosis** with **RV outflow obstruction** and 4) **RVH**. Initially, a shunt can be created surgically to maintain blood supply to the lungs distal to the pulmonary artery stenosis **(66)**. This is usually done by anastomosis of the subclavian artery to the pulmonary artery (Blalock–Taussig shunt). Subsequent surgical treatment is aimed at relieving the outflow obstruction and closing the VSD **(66)**. Long-term complications include RV enlargement and impaired ventricular function leading to reduced exercise capacity, arrhythmias and increased risk of sudden death.

Answers

64. T T T T
65. T T (sometimes known as Eisenmenger's complex) F F T
66. See explanation

67. Regarding classification of cardiomyopathy

    a. What are the three main types of cardiomyopathy?
    b. Which is the most common?
    c. Which is a differential diagnosis of constrictive pericarditis?
    d. Which one can be attributed to alcohol?
    e. Which is associated with sudden death?

68. A young man in his 20s presents to you as his GP for reassurance. He has been experiencing palpitations and is worried that this may be a warning that he might have a heart attack, as his father died suddenly aged 40 years from a 'heart problem'. He is otherwise fit and well. You are about to reassure him, but decide to ask a few more questions and perform an examination

    a. What do you need to exclude?
    b. What features in the history and examination might you look for?

He has not had any pain or episodes of syncope, but on direct questioning says that he is sometimes short of breath. He is not aware of any other relevant family history. On examination, his pulse is 'jerky' and you hear an S3 and S4 as well as a quiet systolic murmur.

    c. What investigations would you request?

ECG is relatively normal, though there is T wave inversion in some of the leads. Echocardiography shows asymmetrical thickening of the septum measuring 30 mm at the widest point.

    d. He wants to know what treatments are available. What do you tell him?

69. A rather grey-looking 65-year-old man hobbles into the cardiology clinic. He sits down and before he starts talking he needs to get his breath back. He tells you that he has become increasingly breathless and tired, and his ankles are swollen. His past medical history includes haemochromatosis diagnosed 13 years ago and diabetes diagnosed last year. On examination, his heart rate is 90 bpm, his JVP is raised 6 cm, and he has peripheral oedema, a 1 cm liver edge and ascites

    a. What type of cardiomyopathy could he have?
    b. investigation would you require to make a diagnosis?

Echocardiography shows that there is no ventricular dilatation or hypertrophy and that the dysfunction is diastolic.

    c. What other key differential diagnosis would you like to exclude?

S3, third heart sound; S4, fourth heart sound

EXPLANATION: CARDIOMYOPATHY

The cardiomyopathies are a collection of disorders of the myocardium, with a broad range of aetiologies and pathologies. In all cases, echocardiography is the investigation of choice as it enables diagnosis and assists in determining prognosis.

Dilated cardiomyopathy is dilatation of the ventricles with reduced ventricular contractile force, resulting in **impaired systolic function**, reduced cardiac output and eventually congestive cardiac failure. It can be familial or acquired through primary myocardial disease such as myocarditis. It is also commonly caused by excess alcohol consumption, and is associated with other systemic conditions such as thiamine deficiency, thyrotoxicosis and haemochromatosis, It presents with symptoms and signs of congestive cardiac failure. **ACE inhibitors**, **beta-blockers** and **spironolactone** are used to palliate symptoms, and a **biventricular pacemaker** can be implanted in cases of ventricular dyssynchrony. Cardiac transplantation is an important option in younger patients.

Hypertrophic cardiomyopathy results from mutations in genes encoding myocardial proteins such as troponin T and tropomyosin. It is inherited in an autosomal dominant manner and has a prevalence of 0.2 per cent. The hypertrophy is often asymmetrical and results in a reduction in the volume of the ventricular cavity. This reduces filling capacity and thereby causes **diastolic dysfunction**. It presents with symptoms of angina, dyspnoea, palpitations and syncope and can cause sudden death. Examination findings include a jerky pulse, a prominent a wave in the JVP, a double apex beath, audible S3 and S4, and a systolic murmur **(68b)**. Patients diagnosed with hypertrophic cardiomyopathy should be advised against participating in competitive sport or sudden strenuous exercise. Myocardial demand can be reduced pharmacologically with **beta-blockers** and/or calcium channel antagonists **(68d)**. **Dual-chamber pacing** or septal ablation is appropriate in those who remain symptomatic **(68d)**.

Restrictive cardiomyopathy is the least common type of cardiomyopathy. It is primarily a **disorder of diastolic function** due to increased rigidity of the myocardium. It can be idiopathic, but is also associated with systemic conditions such as amyloidosis, haemochromatosis, endomyocardial fibrosis, sarcoidosis, and scleroderma. As in dilated cardiomyopathy, it presents with symptoms and signs of heart failure. Echocardiography **(68c)** demonstrates normal systolic function with impaired diastolic filling, atrial dilatation and a speckled or echogenic myocardium, indicative of the underlying aetiology. Treatment is directed at investigating and managing the underlying cause. Atrial fibrillation is common and should be treated with **warfarin**. **ACE inhibitors** help to relieve symptoms by reducing ventricular load.

Answers

67. a – Dilated, hypertrophic (obstructive), restrictive, b – Dilated, c – Restrictive, d – Dilated, e – Hypertrophic
68. a – Hypertrophic cardiomyopathy, b–d – See explanation
69. a – Dilated or restrictive cardiomyopathy, b – Echocardiography is diagnostic, c – Constrictive pericarditis

TREATMENTS

TREATMENTS

A 71-year-old woman presents to her GP following a holiday abroad. She is extremely concerned and reports feeling 'very tired and short of breath during the entire holiday'. She describes several incidences of 'feeling dizzy when climbing stairs or walking around museums', and one occasion when she 'nearly fainted'. She also reports an awareness of her heartbeat, and has presented to the GP mainly because she is worried that her heart is 'missing out beats'. She takes no medication and there is nothing else of note in her history.

1. What is your differential diagnosis?

You examine her and find no peripheral signs of cardiovascular disease; however, her heart rate is 37 bpm. You obtain an ECG.

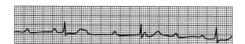

2. What does the ECG show?

3. Which of the following interventions would you recommend?

    a. Atropine
    b. Epinephrine
    c. DC cardioversion
    d. A pacemaker to pace the atrium
    e. A pacemaker to pace the ventricle

4. She is referred to the CCU. Here, she is reassessed by a cardiologist and the decision is made to fit a permanent pacemaker on the following day. Which of the following should be done as part of the normal preoperative workup for this procedure (true or false)?

    a. Insertion of an intravenous cannula, with blood samples taken for full blood count, urea and electrolytes, and clotting
    b. Continuous electrocardiographic monitoring
    c. Written consent for the procedure under a general anaesthetic
    d. Insertion of a temporary pacing wire
    e. Prophylactic flucloxacillin and benzylpenicillin on the evening before the operation

5. List the main risks of the procedure that you would mention when obtaining her consent for the operation

AV, atrioventricular

EXPLANATION: PERMANENT PACEMAKERS

These are relatively small devices that generate **impulses** from a power source, which is usually sited inferior to the left clavicle. Travelling down pacing wires to the electrode tip(s), the impulses initiate depolarization of the myocardium. This is an essential device in patients who have symptomatic disturbances of the conductive pathways of the heart.

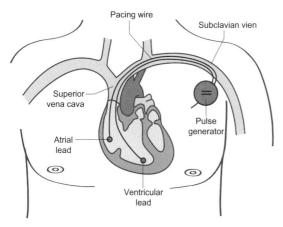

Dual chamber pacemaker

Indicators for a pacemaker include complete AV block, persistant AV block after anterior MI, Mobitz type II AV block, symptomatic bradycardia, drug-resistant tachyarrhythmia, or drug-induced bradycardia due to treatment of tachyarrhythmia. Each pacemaker carries an international three or four letter **code** giving information about: 1) the site of *pacing* e.g. atrial (A), ventricular (V) or dual chamber (D); 2) the site of *sensing* (most pacemakers work only when they are needed); 3) the *response* to sensing; and 4) an additional R can be added if the pulse generator is 'rate adaptive'.

In routine practice, the typical implanted device is a **DDDR**, which can automatically sense and pace as necessary. An exception is patients with permanent atrial fibrillation who receive a VVIR device. Pacemakers can be programmed and their batteries tested through the skin. They need checking every six to twelve months, but have a lifespan of 7–15 years. In our 71-year-old woman, the indication for pacing is complete AV block. She would be most likely to receive a DDD±R pacemaker.

Pacemakers are usually implanted under a local anaesthetic. Flucloxacillin and benzylpenicillin are the preferred prophylactic antibiotics; they have a short half-life and are given just before the procedure begins. **Postoperative care** includes prophylactic antibiotics at 1 and 6 hours, managing pain, checking the wound for bleeding, haematoma, infection or dehiscence, checking that the resting heart rate is within 6 bpm of its setting, performing CXR, booking a pacemaker check-up appointment and giving the patient a pacemaker ID card (contains pacemaker details). The patient should be advised **(6)** to see her GP if the wound becomes hot, red or sore, and not to drive for 1 week or undertake heavy lifting with her left arm. She should not undergo any MRI scans in the future, and should always carry her pacemaker ID card.

Answers

1. LV failure, pulmonary embolism, ectopic beats, atrial fibrillation, bradycardia, sick sinus syndrome or hypothyroidism
2. Third degree AV block/complete heart block
3. a (short-term treatment for symptomatic bradycardia), e (best long-term solution)
4. T T F F F
5. Bleeding, punctured lung, infection, scar, feeling it under her skin, antibiotic reaction

A relatively fit 71-year-old man arrives on your ward for elective cardiac surgery. Over recent months, he has been getting chest pain on exertion that has become more frequent. He was prescribed GTN two months ago and that relieved his pain for the first few weeks; however, the angina has been getting worse and now occurs at rest. He has a past history of smoking but gave up 19 years ago, his hypertension is well controlled on bendrofluazide and he is also on aspirin and a statin. He is eager to have the operation, as his father and brother both had an MI before the age of 60 years. His angiogram was reviewed a few weeks ago in clinic and shows severe stenosis of the left main stem coronary artery.

6. (a) What are his risk factors for cardiovascular disease and (b) what operation might he have come in for?

7. Answer his following questions as short-answer questions

    a. What are the complications of cardiopulmonary bypass?
    b. Can you describe the operation?
    c. What are the more common or dangerous risks and complications of cardiac surgery?
    d. What are the differences between leg vein and internal mammary artery grafts?
    e. How quickly can he get back to activities like driving and gardening afterwards?

Another patient arrives on the ward for elective surgery. He is 65 years old and has been suffering exertional chest pain and dyspnoea for several years. On examination, his pulse is 80 bpm and regular but slow rising in character, and his BP is 150/70 mmHg. You listen to his heart and there is quiet S2; you also hear a harsh ejection systolic murmur at the right external sternal edge that radiates to the carotids.

8. (a) What is the likely diagnosis? (b) Which other symptom might you ask about in the history? (c) What operation has he come for? (d) What preoperative assessments will he have had?

9. You discuss with him the options for valve replacement. Answer his following questions as short-answer questions

    a. What are the main types of tissue valve?
    b. What are mechanical valves like?
    c. What are the advantages and disadvantages of tissue versus prosthetic valves?

CABG, coronary artery bypass graft; IHD, ischaemic heart disease; S2, second heart sound; PTCA, percutaneous transluminal coronary angioplasty

EXPLANATION: CARDIAC SURGERY

Cardiac surgery is mainly used for **bypass grafting**, **valve disease** or **congenital heart disorders**. Surgically correctable complications of MI include repair of mitral valve leak, repair of ventricular or septal rupture and ablation of an arrhythmic focus. Mortality is 5–30 per cent.

Cardiac surgery is major surgery with 5–30 per cent mortality. During surgery the heart is stopped and blood is pumped by the cardiac bypass machine. Heparin is added to reduce clotting, and complications therefore include bleeding. Red blood cell heamolysis and platelet destruction occur due to the mechanical shearing forces. Complement system activation results in increased capillary permeability, inflammation and haemodilution leading to the development of oedema. Stroke occurs in 1–2 per cent of patients **(7a)**. Other general perioperative complications include hypertension, MI, arrhythmias, hypoxia, hypothermia and renal failure **(7c)**.

Preoperative work-up includes ECG, echocardiography and sometimes Doppler echocardiography. General assessment of fitness for surgery includes ventricular, pulmonary and renal function tests as well as full blood count, clotting profile and blood cross-match **(8d)**.

Indications for **CABG** include coronary artery disease that is unlikely to be more safely treated by PTCA. Lesions that are best dealt with by CABG include left main stem lesions or complex calcified proximal lesions in multiple arteries. The internal mammary artery or long saphenous vein is used to bypass the stenosis **(7b)**. 85–90 per cent of patients are relieved of the symptoms of angina. 50 per cent of vein grafts and 90 per cent of artery grafts are patent at 10 years, however artery grafts are often associated with chest wall numbness **(7d)**.

Indications for **valve replacement** include severe stenosis and pressure gradient across a valve in a patient who is symptomatic. Complications of **prosthetic valves** include haemolysis, structural failure, infective endocarditis and systemic embolism. **Tissue valves** (homografts or xenografts, usually pig **(9a)**) have the advantage that anticoagulation is not required **(9c)** except for during the first three months postoperatively; however, they are prone to failure after 8–12 years **(9c)**. **Mechanical valves** such as the St Jude double tilting disc, ball and cage, and porcelain valves **(9b)** are more durable **(9c)** and are therefore frequently used in young patients with a long life expectancy. They have the disadvantage of the need for life-long anticoagulation and they carry a higher risk of bacterial endocarditis **(9c)**; antibiotic prophylaxis is therefore indicated before surgical or dental procedures.

Answers

6. a – Smoking, hypertension, high cholesterol and family history, b – PTCA or CABG
7. a–d – See explanation, e – Drive after 1 month, start gentle exercise, gardening by 3 months
8. a – Aortic stenosis, b – Syncope, c – Aortic valve replacement, d – See explanation
9. See explanation

10. Regarding drugs used in the treatment of hypertension, answer true or false

a. Diuretics are a first-line treatment in hypertension

b. Beta-blockers are more effective in younger patients

c. Angiotensin II antagonists can be used if angiotensin-converting enzyme inhibitors cause a dry cough

d. Calcium channel antagonists may cause angio-oedema

e. Patients with asthma and hypertension should be given beta-blockers

11. Which of the following drugs used to treat angina have been proven to reduce mortality?

a. Nitrates

b. Statins

c. Angiotensin-coverting enzyme inhibitors

d. Beta-blockers

e. Aspirin

12. Regarding the treatment of heart failure, answer true or false

a. Nitrates work by increasing venous return to the heart

b. Inotropic agents have been proven to reduce mortality from heart failure

c. Beta-blockers are contraindicated in chronic heart failure

d. Angiotensin-converting enzyme inhibitors act by reducing preload and afterload on the heart

e. Frusemide may cause hyperkalaemia

13. Regarding the treatment of AF, answer true or false

a. Anticoagulation is usually necessary

b. Rhythm and rate control should be obtained in all cases of atrial fibrillation

c. Digoxin is effective at controlling ventricular rhythm

d. Amiodarone is a potent agent for rhythm control

e. Sotalol is used in paroxysmal atrial fibrillation

AF, atrial fibrillation; ISMN, isosorbide mononitrate

EXPLANATION: EVIDENCE-BASED PHARMACOLOGICAL TREATMENT OF COMMON CARDIOVASCULAR CONDITIONS

Condition	Drug aims	Drug	Example	Trial that tested the class of drug
Hypertension	Diuretics	Thiazides	Bendroflumethiazide	MRC, ALLHAT
	Vasodilators	ACE inhibitors	Ramipril	HOPE
		Angiotensin II antagonists	Losartan	LIFE
		Ca^{2+} channel blockers	Amlodipine	ASCOT
		α-blockers	Doxazosin	
	Negative inotropes/ chronotropes	β-blockers	Bisoprolol	MRC
Ischaemic heart disease	Reduce mortality	Antiplatelet agents	Aspirin	Physicians' Health Study
			Clopidogrel	CURE
			Glycoprotein IIb/IIIa antagonists	TARGET
		ACE inhibitors	Perindopril	HOPE, PROGRESS, EUROPA
		Lipid-lowering agents	Simvastatin	Scandinavian Simvastatin Study, Heart Protection Study
		β-blockers	Atenolol	ASIST
	Reduce symptoms	Nitrates	GTN, ISMN	
		Calcium channel blockers	Amlodipine, diltiazem	
Heart failure	Improve prognosis	ACE inhibitors	Enalapril	CONSENSUS
		Angiotensin II antagonists	Candesartan	CHARM
		β-blockers	Bisoprolol	CIBIS-II
		Aldosterone blockade	Spironolactone	RALES
		Nitrates and hydralazine		V-HeFT, A-HeFT
	Reduce symptoms	Cardiac glycosides	Digoxin	DIG-1
		Loop diuretics	Furosemide	
		Inotropes	Vesnarinone	VEST (showed increased mortality)
AF	Rate control	Cardiac glycosides	Digoxin	DIG-1
		β-blockers	Atenolol	
		Ca^{2+} channel blockers	Verapamil	
	Rhythm control (acute AF)	Anti-arrhythmics	Amiodarone, sotalol	AFFIRM
	Anticoagulation	Coumarins	Warfarin (INR 2–3)	EAFT
		Antiplatelet agents	Aspirin (if warfarin contraindicated)	

Answers

10. T T T F (ACE inhibitors cause angio-oedema) F

11. b, c (HOPE and EUROPA), d, e. Nitrates provide symptomatic relief only

12. F (decrease VR to heart) F F (reduce mortality in chronic heart failure) T F (may cause hypokalaemia)

13. T (about 50 per cent of acute AF lasts >24 to 48 hours, when embolic risk rises, so most clinicians anticoagulate from the outset) F F (rate not rhythm) T T

14. Match the following side effects to the most appropriate drug class

Options

A. Gynaecomastia
B. Gastritis
C. Bleeding
D. Dry cough
E. Thyroid dysfunction
F. Bronchospasm

1. Beta-blockers
2. Warfarin
3. Amiodarone
4. Spironolactone
5. Aspirin
6. Angiotensin-converting enzyme inhibitors

15. Answer the following as true or false

a. Beta-blockers are contraindicated in renal artery stenosis
b. Porphyria is an indication for spironolactone
c. Beta-blockers are suitable only for use in asthmatics
d. Warfarin is contraindicated in patients who are likely to fall often
e. Warfarin is contraindicated in the second trimester of pregnancy
f. Thiazide diuretics are contraindicated in Addison's disease

COPD, chronic obstructive pulmonary disease; HOCM, hypertrophic obstructive cardiomyopathy

EXPLANATION: SIDE EFFECTS OF AND CONTRAINDICATIONS TO COMMON CARDIOVASCULAR DRUGS

Common drugs	Contraindications	Major adverse effects
ACE inhibitors	Renal artery stenosis and aortic stenosis	Dry cough, first-dose hypotension, angio-oedema, hyperkalaemia
Angiotensin II antagonists	Cholestasis (with candesartan)	Hyperkalaemia, postural hypotension
Alpha-blockers	Postural hypotension, micturition syncope	Headache, postural hypotension
Amiodarone	Bradycardia, history of thyroid disease or iodine sensitivity	Thyroid dysfunction, photosensitivity, pulmonary fibrosis
Aspirin	<16 years old (Reye's syndrome), peptic ulcer disease	Gastritis, bleeding, contraindicated in peptic ulcer disease
β-blockers	Asthma and COPD (relative)	Bronchospasm, cold peripheries, bradycardia, rising glucose, rising lipids
Ca^{2+} channel blockers	Cardiogenic shock, severe aortic stenosis	Flushing, fatigue, ankle swelling, postural hypotension
Digoxin	Heart block, HOCM	Bradyarrhythmia, complete heart block
Loop diuretics	Severe liver cirrhosis	Hypokalaemia, postural hypotension, impotence
Nitrates	Hypotension, aortic/mitral stenosis, constrictive pericarditis/tamponade, HOCM, glaucoma	Headache, hypotension
Sotalol	Asthma, peripheral arterial disease, long QT syndrome, torsade de pointes	Bradycardia, hypotension, arrhythmia, cold peripheries, fatigue, insomnia
Spironolactone	Hyperkalaemia, hyponatraemia, Addison's disease, porphyria	Hyperkalaemia, gynaecomastia
Statins	Liver disease	Myositis, deranged liver function
Thiazide diuretics	Hypokalaemia, hyponatraemia, Addison's disease	Dehydration and postural hypotension, hypokalaemia, impotence
Verapamil	SA node block, second-/third-degree heart block	Constipation, hypotension, heart failure
Warfarin (INR 2–3)	Active bleeding, high risk of bleeding (e.g. frequent falls), early pregnancy	Haemorrhage, 1% risk of stroke

Answers

14. A – 4, B – 5, C – 2, D – 6, E – 3, F – 1
15. F F F T F T

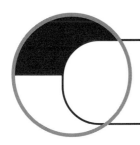

APPENDIX

CHOOSING DRUGS FOR PATIENTS NEWLY DIAGNOSED WITH HYPERTENSION

Abbreviations:
A = ACE inhibitor
(consider angiotonsin-II receptor
antagonist if ACE intolerant)
C = calcium-channel blocker
D = thiazide-type diuretic

Black patients are those of African or
Caribbean descent and not mixed-race,
Asian or Chinese patients

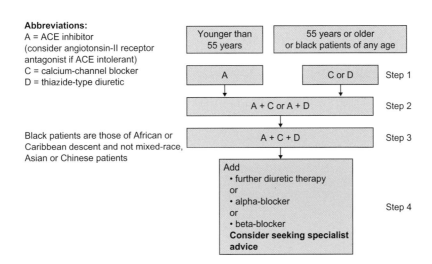

Reproduced from: National Collaborating Centre for Chronic Conditions. *Hypertension: management in adults in primary care: pharmacological update.* London: Royal College of Physicians, 2006. Copyright © 2006 Royal College of Physicians. Reproduced by permission. Also, National Institute for Health and Clinical Excellence (NICE) and the British Hypertention Society (2006) 'Choosing drugs for patients newly diagnosed with hypertension', *Hypertension: management of hypertension in adults in primary care* (Quick reference guide); London: NICE. Available from www.nice.org.uk/page.aspx?o=CG034quickrefguide. Reproduced with permission.

CHARACTERISTICS OF THE THREE MAIN CORONARY SYNDROMES

	Unstable angina	NSTEMI	STEMI
Pathophysiology	Ischaemia without necrosis	Subendocardial infarct	Transmural infarct
Presentation (*not* specific)	Increasing severity and frequency of angina symptoms, partially relieved by GTN	Severe angina pain lasting >20 minutes	Severe chest pain, lasting >30 minutes, nausea, vomiting, sweating, not relieved by GTN
ECG	No ST segment or T wave changes	No ST segment changes T wave inversion may be present	ST elevation or depression: >2 mm in chest leads, >1 mm in limb leads, Q waves, T wave inversion, new left bundle branch block
Thrombolysis status	Not eligible	Not eligible	Thrombolysis indicated, if emergency angiography unavailable
Cardiac biomarkers	Cardiac markers are not raised	More than two-fold increase in serum levels of cardiac proteins Troponin T and I rise within 4–8 hours and remain elevated for 4–7 days Creatine kinase MB rises within 4–8 hours, peaks at 24 hours, returns to normal at 2–3 days	As for NSTEMI

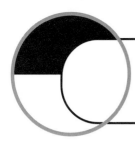

INDEX